CLINICAL DEPRESSION DURING ADDICTION RECOVERY

PROCESS, DIAGNOSIS, AND TREATMENT

EDITED BY

JERRY S. KANTOR

Addiction Recovery Centre
Fort Myers, Florida

Marcel Dekker, Inc.   New York • Basel • Hong Kong

Library of Congress Cataloging-in-Publication Data

Clinical depression during addiction recovery: process, diagnosis,
 and treatment / edited by Jerry S. Kantor.
  p. cm.
 Includes bibliographical references and index.
 ISBN 0-8247-9622-5 (hardcover: alk. paper)
 1. Depression, Mental—Treatment. 2. Recovering addicts—Mental
health. I. Kantor, Jerry S.
 [DNLM: 1. Depressive Disorder—diagnosis. 2. Depressive Disorder—
therapy. 3. Substance Dependence—rehabilitation. WM 171 C6405
1996]
RC537.C558 1996
616.85'27—dc20
DNLM/DLC
for Library of Congress

95-45645
CIP

The publisher offers discounts on this book when ordered in bulk quantities. For more information, write to Special Sales/Professional Marketing at the address below.

This book is printed on acid-free paper.

MARCEL DEKKER, INC.
270 Madison Avenue, New York, New York 10016

Current printing (last digit):
10 9 8 7 6 5 4 3 2 1

PRINTED IN THE UNITED STATES OF AMERICA

To my two beautiful children,
Justin and Jessica

Foreword

> In addition to my other numerous acquaintances, I have one more intimate
> confidant. . . . My depression is the most faithful mistress I have known—no
> wonder, then, that I return the love.
>
> Soren Kierkegaard (1843), *Diapsalmata*

DEPRESSION: A BROAD-SPECTRUM DISORDER

Depressive disorders range from a relatively simple, time-limited dysthymia to a more complicated and enduring bipolar illness with intense
depression. Depression, often characterized by strong feelings of sadness, guilt, worthlessness, and malaise, also can include symptoms that
include sleep disorder, isolation, lack of sexual interest, loss of appetite,
suicidal ideation and suicidal behaviors. Bipolar affect disorder is a
more complex depression that can include psychosis and a wide variety
of other sequelae. There is no single entity that we can call depression.
Instead, depression is best thought of as a broad-spectrum disorder.
This disorder tends to shift perspective toward events past and preclude
interest in the future.

Some depressive episodes can be stimulated by the cessation of
psychoactive drug use. For example, stopping the regular and immoder-
ate use of cocaine can lead to a dysthymic reaction (i.e., anhedonia),
on the one hand, and to acute suicidal behavior, on the other. When
patients first enter treatment for substance-abuse disorders, they often

appear depressed; however, as treatment continues, this depression often begins to remit (e.g., Jaffe and Ciraulo, 1986). The waxing and waning of depression during substance abuse and recovery led clinicians to wonder whether depression causes substance abuse or substance abuse stimulates depression? If substance abuse does stimulate depression, does the depression reside latently, awakened only by the trauma of addiction or, alternatively, can substance abuse give rise to "original" depression? These important questions are rarely addressed. Kantor and his contributors set out to remedy this situation as well as other vexing issues in *Clinical Depression During Addiction Recovery: Processes, Diagnosis, and Treatment.*

DEPRESSION AND SUBSTANCE ABUSE—CART OR HORSE?

Addiction is a very complex and unyielding phenomenon. Recovery from addiction can be as perplexing as addiction. As I mentioned before, while many patients who enter treatment reveal depression that meets diagnostic levels, depression can also emerge after addiction wanes and recovery emerges. This coincidence of depression and substance abuse often led both casual and professional observers to conclude that these patterns represent an enduring addiction motif. These confluent conditions expose themselves regularly as a pattern of comorbidity that is common among patients struggling with addictive disorders (e.g., Weiss et al., 1988). Whenever a substance-abusing patient presents with depression, clinicians must investigate antecedent and consequent events. Is the depression antecedent to the substance-abusing pattern or has the use of psychoactive substances insidiously stimulated depression? When depression precedes substance abuse, a series of possibilities exist to help both patient and provider to understand the complex patterns of substance abuse. However, before discussing some of these treatment considerations, it is very important to remember that for many patients depression actually results from—rather than engenders—the experience of protracted substance abuse. Furthermore, and less well recognized, depression can be stimulated by (1) the recession of addiction, (2) the onset of abstinence, and (3) ongoing tasks of recovery.

This book offers clinicians essential information about recovery-stimulated depression. For example, during recovery and without the object of their addiction, patients often sense that they have lost an important organizing element of their daily life; this loss of control—quite different from the experience of control lost during addiction—can stimulate a depressive episode. Once in recovery and without the object of their addiction to assist in shifting undesirable emotional states, many patients are unable to regulate either their behaviors or their impulses as they have in the past. Under these conditions, feelings of helplessness and dysthymia may be stimulated. Similarly, when some people with addiction stop their pattern of intemperance, they become acutely aware of the painful problems that were stimulated by their excessive behaviors. These experiences often can precipitate painful anxious depression. Diminished self-control, exacerbated by experiencing, first, the losses commonly associated with a substance-abusing lifestyle and its other adverse consequences (e.g., health, social, and vocational problems) and, second, the losses associated with abstinence and recovery, can lead to dysthymia and depression.

THE DYNAMICS OF WITHHOLDING: MEDICATION AND SUBSTANCE-ABUSING PATIENTS

Addiction treatment specialists traditionally assume that recovery should be a ''drug-free'' experience. Too often, this assumption has led to undermedicating patients who require pharmacotherapy. For example, once therapists make the determination—if indeed this is possible—that the primary problem is depression, then it is quite reasonable to medicate patients for their distress. However, unlike patients who suffer only from depression, the substance-abusing patient who is depressed presents special challenges for nonprescribing psychotherapists and pharmacotherapists. In their attempt to assert control, substance-abusing patients often split their treatment providers by withholding information from one of the parties. This dynamic is often misunderstood as simple deceit, sociopathy, or, even worse, intractability.

Maintaining Psychic Inertia: Splitting and Denial

When depressed patients with chronic histories of chemical acting out are confronted by information that challenges their psychological inertia—a world view they have evolved and managed to sustain in the face of many previous interferences that encourage change—they protect their identity by splitting and denying alternatives to the current state of affairs. For the uninitiated, this dynamic is quite similar to how science as a process minimizes anomalous research findings and therefore maintains conceptual stability by protecting its body of knowledge from uncertain alternatives (e.g., Kuhn, 1962).

Responding to Withholding: Problems of Countertransference

Therapists often revere science for its capacity to deny alternative information, but punish patients for engaging in similar behavior. Patients often withhold information from their health providers. When clinicians learn of previously withheld (e.g., denied) material, too often the response is patient punishment (e.g., termination). Although it may appear that patients with addiction are provoking their therapists intentionally by withholding necessary treatment information, they, like many scientists presented with anomalous data, are rather simply protecting their world view and the elements of experience that support such a perspective. Behaving angrily toward patients is an example of countertransference hate (cf. Maltsberger and Buie, 1974; Shaffer, 1994). The usual consequence of this type of therapeutic exchange is for patients to hide even more information or, after experiencing the anger of a treatment provider who experiences patient splitting as personal injury, feel sufficiently helpless and insecure that they terminate treatment. Under these circumstances, a patient-initiated termination appears to confirm the often held clinical view that the patient either was not ready for change or was intractable. More often, however, I think that this termination is the result of clinicians who are unable to tolerate both their own anxiety (e.g., Zetzel, 1949) and the patient's complex affect that is associated with wanting to use psychoactive substances.

CLINICAL INTERVENTIONS: NAVIGATING THE PSYCHOTHERAPY OF AMBIVALENCE AND CHANGE

Substance-abuse treatment specialists have not offered a consistent opinion on the matter of medicating patients while they are using or abusing psychoactive substances. This matter is of major importance when considering the treatment of depressed patients. The conventional wisdom among many treatment providers is to require a period of abstinence before any medication is prescribed. In addition to establishing a clearer representation of a patient in the absence of psychoactive medication that might alter mental status, this strategy has the additional benefit of providing a test of motivation. Patients apparently motivated to change will begin a period of abstention when their caretaker requests it. Apparently unmotivated patients will continue to abuse drugs in spite of their entry into treatment. Nevertheless, both patients who flee into abstinence-directed recovery with little struggle and those who continue to abuse substances excessively represent less than healthy responses to entering substance-abuse treatment. Patients who openly struggle with their pattern of drug use, their ambivalent feelings about change (Shaffer, 1994; Shaffer and Robbins, 1991), and the potential impact of such change on their experience, represent a group of patients who are more likely to achieve their long-term recovery objectives (e.g., Shaffer and LaSalvia, 1992). Even if patients enter treatment ready to begin a period of abstinence, therapists still should examine repeatedly any remaining ambivalence about giving up drug use. Clinicians can then permit newly abstinent patients to experience grief for this separation and loss (Shaffer, 1994; Shaffer and Robbins, 1991). If the frequent and excessive use of psychoactive drugs were not essential in some way, patients would usually give up or change their pattern of drug use without entering treatment (e.g., Shaffer and Jones, 1989).

The problem confronting clinicians who deal with addiction is that most substance-abusing patients who enter treatment are not quite ready for complete abstinence (Shaffer, 1994). These patients usually wish that they did want to stop. Psychotherapists cannot easily distinguish patients who are ready to stop using drugs during treatment from those who are not. This situation is complicated further by evidence revealing that as many as 90% of patients who do stop will resort to using again at some point during their recovery (e.g., Marlatt and Gordon, 1985).

Requiring patients to follow a unilaterally (i.e., clinician) imposed treatment plan instead of negotiating mutual clinical objectives is still another example of countertransference-driven therapy. To assure a shared view of therapy, matters of treatment planning and formulation must be reviewed and renegotiated repeatedly during the course of treatment.

Psychotherapy, Prescription Medicine, and the Value of Illicit Drugs

For many psychiatric patients, entry into treatment brings with it the onset of medication. Psychotropic medicine is designed to alleviate psychological discomfort and pain; in addition, psychoactive medications permit many patients to tolerate intense (and therefore often painful) affect so that they can participate effectively in psychotherapy. When patients in treatment continue to use certain substances, similar to patients taking prescribed medication, they are attenuating painful affect by self-medicating their condition (e.g., Khantzian, 1975). While this situation has many obvious disadvantages (e.g., improper dosage, drug and administration pattern), it does—like substance abuse in general—have the benefit of providing an in vivo test of how various medications have worked in the past and therefore might influence the patient in the future. For example, many patients with attention deficit hyperactivity disorders have been diagnosed by clinicians who carefully assessed their paradoxical reactions to illicit stimulant use (e.g., Khantzian et al., 1984). For depressed patients with substance-abuse disorders, a thorough "cost–benefit" analysis associated with substituting prescribed medication for self-selected medication is required.

Substance Abuse and Affect Regulation

Many substance-abusing patients use psychoactive drugs or other addictive behaviors (e.g., pathological gambling) to regulate painful affect. For example, as a psychostimulant, marijuana can reduce some symptoms of agitated depression by providing concurrent stimulation and perceptual distraction. Low-dose alcohol, as a releasing agent, has the capacity to minimize feelings of inadequacy and energize a dysthymic sense of social competence. In higher doses, alcohol can serve analgesic-like functions and simply paralyze the pain of depression. In every case, however, alcohol is indeed a mood magnifier; therefore we should not be surprised that ultimately patients who treat depression with alcohol experience their suffering as "worse." The stimulating properties of cocaine can directly but fleetingly provide patients with effects similar to those of some antidepressants. Regular or long-term use of cocaine, however, ultimately leaves patients with anergia and anhedonia that encourages them to use the drug repeatedly, perhaps as a method to access the earlier stimulating, antidepressant effect.

Finally, even nonchemical addictions can serve as anodynes for painful depression. For example, McCormick et al. (1984) found that "gambling did seem to act as an antidepressant activity for many subjects who reported periods when their overall mood was very depressed except when they were actively gambling. Gambling was the only activity that seemed capable of energizing them and altering their mood" (p. 217). Ultimately, excessive gambling, like psychostimulants, often leaves users feeling the pain of dysthymia and depression.

THE CENTERPIECE OF PSYCHOTHERAPY WITH ADDICTION: AMBIVALENCE ABOUT SUBSTANCE USE

When treatment specialists are willing to look, substance-abusing patients usually evidence considerable ambivalence about their drug use. This is true even when prescribed medications can provide significant relief from feelings of depression. This ambivalence derives primarily from a user's previous and more positive experiences with drug use and the sense that drugs provide him with the opportunity to manipulate his subjective state independently (Shaffer, 1994). In spite of any recognition that the use of psychoactive substances represents self-destructive patterns of behavior, most patients will admit that they are not ready to give up these drugs. They are not yet ready to stop because, on some level, a part of their being likes what psychoactive drug use does for them. Under these circumstances, clinicians must neither punish nor simply repeatedly discuss drug-using patterns. Therapy must address how these drugs work for each patient, under what conditions these drugs produce the desired or undesired effect(s), what part of a patient's experience is fulfilled by each drug or combination of drugs, and what other activities or alternatives are available to substitute for these effects. Psychotherapists must also recognize that attempting to substitute activities that may be less potent than the illicitly applied drugs is a tall order, since most psychoactive substances produce relatively reliable subjective effects. Substituting less reliable experiences can be frustrating for patients—on occasion, these shifts can stimulate depression. Change is often a very stressful experience and should be considered a potential precursor for the onset of depressive states (Dohwrenwend and Dohwrenwend, 1974). However, once these substitutions and lifestyle revisions are made *and* sustained for an extended period of time, personality shifts do emerge and patients "change" (e.g., Shaffer and Jones, 1989; Vaillant, 1983; Zinberg, 1984).

Kantor has taken on a task of great importance: in this volume the myriad of issues associated with addiction and depression are examined carefully and comprehensively. The contributors to this volume consider the major factors associated with the synergy between depression and addiction. Treatments are described from both pharmacological and therapeutic perspectives. Given the sheer prevalence of complex clinical issues that emerge when depressed patients with addiction participate in treatment, this book is an important contribution to the clinical literature and should be on the reading list of every addiction treatment specialist.

Howard J. Shaffer, Ph.D., C.A.S.
Division on Addictions, Harvard
Medical School, Boston, and
Cambridge Hospital, Cambridge,
Massachusetts

REFERENCES

Dohwrenwend, B. S., and Dohwrenwend, B. P. (eds.) (1974). *Stressful Life Events: Their Nature and Effects.* New York: John Wiley and Sons.

Jaffe, J. H., and Ciraulo, D. A. (1986). Alcoholism and depression. In R. E. Meyer (ed.), *Psychopathology and Addictive Disorders.* New York: Guilford Press, pp. 293–320.

Khantzian, E. J. (1975). Self-selection and progression in drug dependence. *Psychiatry Digest,* 36:19–22.

Khantzian, E. J., Gawin, F., Kleber, H. D., and Riordan, C. E. (1984). Methylphenidate (ritalin) treatment of cocaine dependence—a preliminary report. *Journal of Substance Abuse Treatment, 1:*107–112.

Kuhn, T. S. (1962). *The Structure of Scientific Revolutions.* Chicago: University of Chicago Press.

Maltsberger, J. T., and Buie, D. (1974). Countertransference hate in the treatment of suicidal patients. *Archives of General Psychiatry, 30:*625–633.

Marlatt, G. A., and Gordon, J. R. (eds.) (1985). *Relapse Prevention: Maintenance Strategies in the Treatment of Addictive Behaviors.* New York: Guilford Press.

McCormick, R. A., Russo, A. M., Ramirez, L. F., and Taber, J. I. (1984). Affective disorders among pathological gamblers seeking treatment. *American Journal of Psychiatry, 141:*215–218.

Shaffer, H. J. (1994). Denial, ambivalence and countertransference hate. In J. D. Levin and Weiss, R.(eds.), *Alcoholism: Dynamics and Treatment: The Essential Papers.* Northdale, N.J.: Jason Aronson, pp. 421–437.

Shaffer, H. J. (1992). The psychology of stage change: the transition from addiction to recovery. In J. Lowinson et al. (eds.), *Comprehensive Textbook of Substance Abuse.* Baltimore: Williams & Wilkins.

Shaffer, H. J., and LaSalvia, T. (1992). Patterns of substance use among methadone maintenance patients: indicators of outcome. *Journal of Substance Abuse Treatment, 9(2):*143–147.

Shaffer, H. J., and Jones, S. B. (1989). *Quitting Cocaine: The Struggle Against Impulse.* Lexington: Lexington Books.

Shaffer, H. J., and Robbins, M. (1991). Manufacturing multiple meanings of addiction: time-limited realities. *Contemporary Family Therapy: An International Journal, 13(5):*387–404.

Vaillant, G. (1983). *The Natural History of Alcoholism.* Cambridge, Mass.: Harvard University Press.

Weiss, R. D., Mirin, S. M., Griffin, M, L., and Michael, J. L. (1988). A comparison of alcoholic and nonalcoholic drug abusers. *Journal of Studies on Alcohol, 49:*510–515.

Zetzel, E. (1949). Anxiety and the capacity to bear it. *International Journal of Psychoanalysis, 30:*1–12.

Zinberg, N. E. (1984). *Drug, Set, and Setting: The Basis for Controlled Intoxicant Use.* New Haven: Yale University Press.

Preface

The purpose of *Clinical Depression During Addiction Recovery* is to help clinicians recognize and effectively treat the different types of depression that may occur during early recovery from addiction.

The book begins with a review of the current theoretical constructs regarding depression in patients recovering from a broad range of addictions. Psychological, social, and biological perspectives are first considered, providing the reader with a clear rationale for the clinical applications of diagnosis and treatment that follow later in the book.

Almost everyone who enters recovery will experience feelings of depression at some point during the first year. Some people experience only mild depression that gradually resolves with time and continued participation in a recovery program. Others experience moderate depression that requires specific psychological treatment. Still others become severely depressed and require antidepressant medication. This book guides clinicians through the differential diagnosis and treatment of these different types of depression. (Note that alcohol and drug intoxication, as well as withdrawal, can produce organic affective disorder, a state often indistinguishable from major depressive disorder.)

Fortunately, most patients see a clearing of affective symptoms after several drug-free weeks. Clinicians must be aware of these phenomena to avoid inappropriate treatment with antidepressants. On the other hand, the clinician must carefully weigh the patient's personal psychiatric history and family history and the longitudinal course of the symptoms during withdrawal so as not to withhold treatment with antidepressants from the minority of patients who require it at the very outset.

Most patients' depression will clear without any specific treatment after a drug-free period of several weeks, only to return at some point during the first few months of sobriety. This occurs because during treatment the patient must cope with many losses. Every patient who has entered recovery gives up his addictive behavior as a way to change his mood. Before this, whenever he was upset or faced with difficulties, he could turn to that addictive behavior as a mood changer. Not being able to use this way out represents a profound loss. Because of denial, by the time a patient with addictive disease seeks treatment his life is in a shambles, confronting him with multiple serious losses. His finances are usually depleted, his important relationships are severely strained, his job is in jeopardy, and he may have legal problems. During early recovery, the hope that accepting sobriety will magically solve all these problems eventually gives way to reality.

Almost everyone will experience some form of clinical depression. The clinician's challenge is to identify the specific type of depression present and the treatment approach most likely to work. This book will arm therapists for this challenge with a theoretical framework and practical approaches for accurate diagnosis and successful treatment.

The book will appeal to addictionologists, psychiatrists, psychologists, social workers, counselors, clergy, and anyone involved in the treatment of people entering recovery from a broad range of addictions.

I would like to thank the many colleagues and teachers who took the time to sit down and review this manuscript and give me their feedback and ideas. I would like specifically to thank Dr. Robert Michels, Dr. David Liebling, David Peer, A.C.S.W., L.C.S.W., Judy Tritel, M.A., L.M.H.C., Chris Seavey, M.A., L.M.H.C., C.A.P., N.C.A.C.I.I., Rose Thorn, Psy.D., Dr. Jonathan Shimshoni, Dr. Robert Willig, and Dr. Martin Keller. I would also like to thank Margel Smith for tireless efforts at coordinating and organizing communication between the contributors and the editor. In addition, I would like to thank June Smith and Pat Rossback for their help in typing and preparing the document. Lastly, I thank Mona Moffet for her suggestions and help in improving my syntax and grammar.

Jerry S. Kantor

Contents

Contributors

Willa Bernhard, Ph.D.   Instructor, Department of Psychiatry, Cornell University Medical College, New York, New York

Joseph R. Calabrese, M.D.   Director, Mood Disorders Program, Vice Chairman, Clinical Affairs, Associate Professor of Psychiatry, University Hospitals of Cleveland and Case Western Reserve University School of Medicine, Cleveland, Ohio

Sabrina Cherry, M.D.   Assistant Clinical Professor of Psychiatry, Department of Psychiatry, Columbia University College of Physicians and Surgeons and Presbyterian Hospital, New York, New York

Norman Cotterell, Ph.D.   Assistant Director of Education, Center for Cognitive Therapy, University of Pennsylvania, Philadelphia, Pennsylvania

Thomas J. D'Zurilla, Ph.D.   Associate Professor, Department of Psychology, State University of New York at Stony Brook, Stony Brook, New York

Mark Fulton, M.D. Department of Psychiatry, Dallas Veterans Affairs Medical Center and University of Texas Southwestern Medical School, Dallas, Texas

Michael Holloman, M.D. Department of Psychiatry, Dallas Veterans Affairs Medical Center and University of Texas Southwestern Medical School, Dallas, Texas

Patricia Isbell, M.D. Department of Psychiatry, Dallas Veterans Affairs Medical Center and University of Texas Southwestern Medical School, Dallas, Texas

Jerry S. Kantor, M.D. Medical Director, Addiction Recovery Centre, Fort Myers, Florida

Mary J. Kujawa, M.D., Ph.D. Assistant Professor of Psychiatry and Associate Residency Training Director, Department of Psychiatry, University Hospitals of Cleveland and Case Western Reserve University School of Medicine, Cleveland, Ohio

Raymond W. Lam, M.D., F.R.C.P.(C) Associate Professor, Department of Psychiatry, University of British Columbia and Vancouver Hospital and Health Sciences Centre, Vancouver, British Columbia, Canada

David S. Liebling, M.D. Director, Center for Stress Recovery, Cleveland Veterans Administration Medical Center, Brecksville, Ohio, and Assistant Professor, Department of Psychiatry, Case Western Reserve University School of Medicine, Cleveland, Ohio

John C. Markowitz, M.D. Associate Professor of Clinical Psychiatry, Payne Whitney Clinic, Cornell University Medical College, New York, New York

Barbara J. Mason, Ph.D. Associate Professor and Director of the Division of Substance Abuse, Department of Psychiatry, University of Miami School of Medicine, Miami, Florida

Timothy I. Mueller, M.D. Assistant Professor and Director of Alcohol and Drug Treatment Services, Department of Psychiatry and Human Behavior, Brown University School of Medicine and Butler Hospital, Providence, Rhode Island

Arthur M. Nezu, Ph.D.   Professor and Chair, Department of Clinical and Health Psychology, Medical College of Pennsylvania and Hahnemann University, Philadelphia, Pennsylvania

Christine Maguth Nezu, Ph.D.   Associate Professor, Department of Clinical and Health Psychology, and Associate Dean for Research, School of Health Sciences and Humanities, Medical College of Pennsylvania and Hahnemann University, Philadelphia, Pennsylvania

Raymond L. Ownby, M.D., Ph.D.   Resident in Psychiatry, Department of Psychiatry, University of Miami School of Medicine, Miami, Florida

Frederick Petty, M.D., Ph.D.   Professor and Medical Director, Mental Health Clinic, Dallas Veterans Affairs Medical Center and University of Texas Southwestern Medical School, Dallas, Texas

Jami L. Rothenberg   Doctoral Candidate, Department of Clinical and Health Psychology, Medical College of Pennsylvania and Hahnemann University, Philadelphia, Pennsylvania

1

Clinical Depression During Addiction Recovery: An Overview

Jerry S. Kantor
Addiction Recovery Centre, Fort Myers, Florida

I. INTRODUCTION

An enormous number of people suffer from addictions. Recent prospective epidemiological studies estimate the 1 year prevalence rate for combined alcoholism and substance abuse to be 9.4% of the population, or approximately 15.1 million people (1). If we consider addictions to sex, gambling, and other addictive behaviors, the number is significantly larger.

Washton and Boundy (2) estimate that 14 million to 16 million Americans attend nearly 500,000 self-help groups pursuing recovery from addiction to drugs, alcohol, sex, gambling, and other similar behaviors. Inasmuch as only a small number of addicted patients seek self-help groups, the actual number of people with addictions is much larger.

Unfortunately, almost everyone who enters recovery will at some point experience significant feelings of depression. Most will use the same words, ''I feel depressed,'' so the challenge to the clinician is to identify the specific type of depression and to institute the appropriate treatment.

Some patients experience only a mild depression that gradually resolves with time and continued participation in a recovery program. Drug and alcohol counselors and Alcoholics Anonymous (AA) sponsors have long known that patients often begin to feel better as they attend more of the AA or self-help meetings appropriate for their addiction.

However, some patients continue to attend meetings hoping to feel better, only to become more discouraged and despondent. A significant number simply withdraw and stop attending meetings altogether.

II.   WHY ARE INDIVIDUALS ENTERING RECOVERY FROM ADDICTION ESPECIALLY SUSCEPTIBLE TO DEPRESSIONS?

Patients in early recovery are often psychologically and socially unprepared for the many stresses they will face. In addition, some are biologically vulnerable to more severe forms of depression. As if these reasons were not enough, those individuals addicted to drugs and alcohol may experience exaggerated depressive feelings during intoxication or withdrawal.

Every patient who enters recovery gives up using addictive behavior as a way to change moods. Previously, any time he was upset or faced with difficulties, he could turn to that addictive behavior as a mood changer. Although this was not a constructive solution, it worked. Not being able to use this way out represents a profound loss.

In addition, because of denial, by the time patients with addictive disease seek treatment, their lives are in shambles, confronting them with multiple serious losses. Finances are usually depleted, important relationships are severely strained, work is in jeopardy, and often there are legal problems as well.

During early recovery, the hope that accepting sobriety will magically solve all these problems eventually gives way to reality. Faced with these severe losses, anyone is likely to feel overwhelmed and have difficulty coping.

If the patient's coping mechanisms are impaired, he is likely to react even more strongly. If depression is the primary symptom, this abnormal reaction constitutes an adjustment disorder with depressed mood. Most patients with addictive disease have abnormal coping mechanisms. Many have grown up in dysfunctional families with no positive role models.

The data available on the influence of dysfunctional family life on the future coping abilities of addicted patients come mainly from studies of adult children of alcoholics. Patients who have grown up in nonalcoholic dysfunctional families are likely to have similar coping difficulties. A study comparing alcoholic dysfunctional families with dysfunctional families without an alcoholic member found no significant differences (3).

Yet there is a large body of literature suggesting that adult children of alcoholics have long-term difficulties with social and psychological functioning. Studies have shown patterns of withdrawals from conflict (4), problems with trust, intimacy, and feelings of responsibility and self-esteem (5–8).

Other studies of adults who grew up in alcoholic families demonstrated role confusion (9), decreased communicative skills (10), poor verbal ability, impulsive behavior (11), and a greater likelihood of marital discord (12).

Two reviews using large community samples to compare adult children of alcoholics with controls (13, 14) revealed some discrepancies. Nonetheless, both these controlled studies demonstrated an association between growing up in an alcoholic home and having psychiatric symptoms in adulthood. These studies extend a literature based mainly on descriptive material or studies of fairly small samples.

An individual with addictive disease who grew up in a dysfunctional family will be less able to cope with the stresses of early sobriety. Some of these addictive patients will develop an adjustment disorder with depressed mood. Because of their poorly developed coping mechanisms, they will develop depressive symptoms out of proportion to the demands of the stresses they are facing.

There is a general consensus that the major affective disorders have strong genetic underpinnings (15). Although the major depressive syndromes clearly have a genetic component, identical twins, who have identical genes, are often discordant for depression. This finding suggests that the genetic propensity to depression is not by itself sufficient to cause the illness. Some form of environmental perturbation also seems necessary.

In fact, the latest data in behavioral genetics provide an "unheralded window on the environment" (16). Behavioral genetics provides a chance to study at-risk populations to learn more about environmental contributions.

A recent large study of female/female twin pairs of known zygosity attempted to develop an integrated model to predict vulnerability to depression (17). Of all the variables in Kendler's model, "a recent stressful life event was the most powerful risk factor for major depression."

There is a growing body of literature that associates life events with the onset of major depressive and bipolar disorders. In these individuals, severe life stresses appear to unleash biologically predisposed serious depression. One would expect that even modest stress would elicit a severe response in patients with impaired coping mechanisms. This response is likely to activate any dormant biological vulnerabilities.

Because most addictive patients are facing moderate-to-severe stress during early recovery and have impaired coping mechanisms, they are at high risk for manifesting whatever genetic vulnerabilities they carry.

One careful review demonstrates that life events are more closely associated with the first episode of major depression than with later episodes (18). Post went on to describe a mechanism through which the environment could transduce a change in the genetic makeup of an individual, making him more susceptible to future episodes of depression. This possibility argues strongly for careful, accurate diagnosis and treatment as early as possible during the patient's depressive illness.

III. SOME FORMS OF ADDICTIONS HAVE A SPECIAL ASSOCIATION WITH DEPRESSIVE SYMPTOMS

Sexual addictions are highly associated with depression. In one all-male study, 95% of the sample met Diagnostic and Statistical Manual of Mental Disorders (DSM) III-R criteria for dysthymic disorder, and 55% met the criteria for major depressive disorder (19). Kafka was so impressed with the successful antidepressant treatment of nonparaphilic sexual addictions in men that he conceptualized these behaviors as "sexual dysregulation disorders associated with a primary mood disorder" (20).

Likewise, pathological gambling is highly associated with depression. In two studies, the association was larger than 70% of the sample, n = 50 and n = 25 respectively (21, 22). Roy and colleagues found significantly more undesirable life events during the 6 months before the onset of depression in their sample of pathological gamblers: n = 14 depressed gamblers versus 41 controls (23).

Nicotine dependence, perhaps the most prevalent of all addictions, is also associated with depression. Breslau and colleagues compared nicotine dependent (20%) with nondependent smokers. The dependent group had a higher incidence of major depression and anxiety disorders (24). It has also been reported that having a history of major depression reduces the chances of success in cessation of smoking. "Smokers with a history of major depressive disorder, although not depressed at the time, failed to cease smoking at nearly twice the rate of those free of such a history" (25).

Glassman also notes that for those with a history of depression, it is harder to stop smoking. There is a higher rate of relapse and an increase of depressive episodes during smoking cessation. He adds that pretreatment with antidepressants may be helpful in this subgroup (26).

During intoxication and withdrawal, alcoholic patients can develop depressive symptoms indistinguishable from major depressive disorder. This organic affective disorder usually clears after 2 to 3 weeks of sobriety.

Cocaine-addicted patients also experience intense depressive symptoms during withdrawal that often clear up after 1 or 2 drug-free weeks. Clinicians must be aware of these phenomena to avoid inappropriate treatment with antidepressants. It is important for the clinician to identify the specific type of depression in each patient so the appropriate treatment can be offered.

Not only are depressed patients more likely to relapse to use, they are in emotional pain. Patients with severe forms of depression are at risk for suicide. In a study of 50 alcoholics who actually completed suicide, the authors identified seven nonacute associated features. The most prevalent factor was depression. "Whether as a complication of alcoholism or occurring alone, it is the single most contributory factor to suicide" (27). The authors found that 58% of their patients who completed suicide had comorbid major depressive disorder. In a previous publication, Murphy identified depression in nearly three out of four of the subjects who completed suicide (28).

Educating clinicians to recognize and treat major depression can reduce the frequency of suicide (29). This book was written to enable clinicians to better recognize and effectively treat the types of depression their patients may experience during early recovery from addiction.

To that end, Clinical Depression During Addiction Recovery is organized as follows: Subsequent to this chapter's overview, Chapter 2 outlines the differential diagnosis of depression during recovery. Chapters 3 through 8 are arranged as miniature treatment manuals for each of the common subtypes of depression that most often present themselves to the clinician who treats those patients in recovery.

The next three chapters (9, 10, and 11) discuss the research-driven approaches to psychotherapy for depression and are also arranged as miniature treatment manuals.

In Chapter 2, Dr. Leibling guides the reader as delineated above to orient clinicians to DSM-IV. This will provide the reader with the necessary information to arrive at an accurate diagnosis. For those who are already familiar with DSM-IV, a simple reading of the text will be sufficient. The charts and diagrams can be used as references, and the useful "decision tree" serves as a thought exercise for even the seasoned clinician.

For those who are not as familiar with DSM-IV, I would suggest that they read the text, review the "decision tree," and then study the criteria given in the charts. At that point, it would be helpful to read the text once more.

Readers who are new to the DSM classification system should seek consultation to assist in the diagnosis of their patients. Also, there are many outside readings available to anyone wanting to learn more about the DSM-IV. A series of books published by the American Psychiatric Association Press is especially helpful in this area.

The following six chapters (3 through 8) are, as noted above, essentially miniature treatment manuals for specific treatment approaches to the various depressive subtypes. Each chapter briefly reviews diagnoses and the theoretical underpinnings for current treatment recommendations. The chapters conclude with a hands-on outline for clinical treatment.

In Chapter 3, Dr. Bernhard discusses the treatment for adjustment disorder with depressed mood, whereas in Chapter 4, Dr. Mueller discusses the treatment for major depressive disorder. Drs. Ownby and Mason discuss the treatment for dysthymia in Chapter 5. The treatment for bipolar disorder is the subject of discussion by Drs. Kujawa and Calabrese in Chapter 6.

In Chapter 7, the treatment for organic mood disorder is discussed by Drs. Hollomon, Isbell, Fulton, and Petty. Dr. Lam discusses the treatment for seasonal affective disorder in Chapter 8.

The final three chapters (9, 10, 11) acquaint the reader with the research-driven psychotherapies directed to the treatment of depression. Each begins with a brief review of theoretical constructs and a literature review, then provides a mini treatment manual. In Chapter 9, Dr. Cotterell discusses the cognitive therapy of depression during addiction recovery. Drs. Cherry and Markowitz discuss the use of interpersonal psychotherapy in Chapter 10. The final chapter, 11, presents Drs. Arthur Nezu, Christine Nezu, D'Zurilla, and Rothenberg in a discussion of the use of problem-solving therapy in the treatment of depression during addiction recovery.

When faced with a depressed patient in recovery, the clinician may read Chapter 1 for an overview, followed by Chapter 2 to assist him in arriving at an accurate diagnosis, and then proceed to the appropriate treatment chapters.

Clinical educators will find this text extremely helpful as well, for each chapter can stand alone as a useful course outline on the various subjects.

I am indeed fortunate to have been associated with this dedicated and intelligent group of contributors, each of whom has taken his subject seriously. I believe that as you read through this book, you will join me in commending them on their fine work.

Like them, I fervently hope that our patients will be the ultimate beneficiaries of the more effective clinical management made possible by this text.

REFERENCES

1. D. A. Regier, W. E. Nairow, D. S. Rae, R. W. Manderscheid, B. Z. Locke, F. K. Goodwin, *Arch. Gen. Psychiatry 50:*85–94 (1993).
2. A. B. Washton, D. Boundy, *Willpower's Not Enough,* Harper and Row, New York, 1989, p. 7.
3. M. Rubio-Stipec, H. Bird, G. Canino, M. Bravo, M. Alegria, *J. Stud. Alcohol, 52:*78 (1991).
4. R. M. Cork, *The Forgotten Children: A Study of Children with Alcoholic Parents,* Alcoholism and Drug Research Foundation, Toronto 1969.
5. C. Black, S. F. Bucky, S. Wilder-Padilla, *Int. J. Addictions 21:*213 (1986).
6. T. L. Cermak, S. Brown, *Int. J. Group Psychother. 32:*375 (1982).
7. S. Beletsis, S. Brown, *J. Addiction Health 2:*187–203 (1981).
8. C. B. Cutter, H. S. G. Cutter, *J. Studies Alcohol 48:*29 (1987).
9. P. M. Ward, *J. Social Psychol. 115:*237 (1981).
10. C. Carter, T. H. Nochajski, K. E. Leonard, H. T. Blane, *Br. J. Addiction 85:*1157 (1990).
11. F. Schulsinger, J. Knop, D. W. Goodwin, T. W. Teasdale, U. Mikkelsen, *Arch. Gen. Psychiatry 43:*755 (1986).
12. D. A. Parker, T. C. Harford, *J. Studies Alcohol 49:*306 (1988).
13. S. F. Greenfield, M. S. Swartz, L. R. Landerman, L. K. George, *Am. J. Psychiatry 150:*608–613 (1993).
14. R. Mathew, W. H. Wilson, D. G. Blazer, L. K. George, *Am. J. Psychiatry 150:*793–800 (1993).
15. R. Michels, P. M. Marzuk, *N. Engl. J. Med. 329:*552–560 (1993).
16. D. Reiss, R. Plomin, E. M. Hetherington, *Am. J. Psychiatry 148:*283–291.
17. K. S. Kendler, R. C. Kessler, M. C. Neale, A. C. Heath, L. J. Eaves, *Am. J. Psychiatry 150:*8 (1993).
18. R. M. Post, *Am. J. Psychiatry 149:*999–1010 (1992).
19. M. P. Kafka, R. Prentky, *J. Clin. Psychiatry 53:*351 (1992).
20. M. P. Kafka, *J. Clin. Psychiatry 52:*60 (1991).
21. R. A. McCormick, A. M. Russo, L. F. Ramirez, J. I. Taber, *Am. J. Psychiatry 141:*215 (1984).

22. R. D. Linden, H. G. Pope, J. M. Jonas, *J. Clin. Psychiatry 47:*201 (1986).
23. A. Roy, R. Custer, V. Lorenz, M. Linnoila, *Acta Psychiatr. Scand. 77:*163 (1988).
24. N. Breslau, M. M. Kilbey, P. Adreski, *Arch. Gen. Psychiatry 48:*1069 (1991).
25. A. H. Glassman, F. Stetner, P. S. Walsh Raizman, J. L. Pleiss, T. B. Cooper, L. S. Cokey, *J.A.M.A. 259:*2863 (1988).
26. A. H. Glassman, *Am. J. Psychiatry 150:*546 (1993).
27. G. E. Murphy, R. D. Wetzel, E. Robins, L. McEvoy, *Arch. Gen. Psychiatry 49:*459–463 (1992).
28. G. E. Murphy, J. W. Armstrong, S. L. Hermek, J. R. Fischer, W. W. Clendenin, *Arch. Gen. Psychiatry 36:*65–69 (1979).
29. W. Rutz, L. Von Knorring, J. Walinder, *Acta Psychiatr. Scand. 80:*151–154 (1989).

2

Differential Diagnosis of Depression and Addictive Disorders

David S. Liebling

Center for Stress Recovery, Cleveland Veterans Administration
Medical Center, Brecksville, Ohio, and
Case Western Reserve University School of Medicine,
Cleveland, Ohio

I. INTRODUCTION

Every clinician who treats patients with addictive disorders has observed the frequent occurrence of depressive signs and symptoms (dss) (17). These can occur during periods of drug use or drug withdrawal or during periods of sobriety. In one study of 501 patients seeking treatment for alcohol and drug problems, 19.9% met criteria for current major depression (19). In other studies the percentage of addicted patients who met criteria for major depression was as high as 67% (6). Yet, it is also clear that in the weeks immediately following sobriety fewer and fewer of these patients continue to meet criteria for major depression (6, 19). Several diagnostic questions arise from the co-occurrence of dss and addictive disorders: (a) Are the dss simply an expected manifestation of drug use or withdrawal? (b) Do the dss represent a separate comorbid disorder? (c) What strategies can be employed to facilitate the process of differential diagnosis?

This chapter will address the aforementioned questions. First, there is an examination of a decision tree that can serve as a template for differential diagnosis. Next, there is a detailed discussion of psychopathology and diagnostic criteria of DSM-IV categories of substance intoxication, substance withdrawal, substance-induced mood disorders, major depressive disorder, bipolar disorder, seasonal affective disorder, and dysthymic disorder. Finally, there is a consideration of which specific substances are correlated with dss and DSM-IV syndromes.

Let us first consider the process of differential diagnosis. A decision-tree format can be helpful in highlighting key characteristics that differentiate one diagnostic category from another. Figure 1 depicts a rational process of dealing with dss that occur in temporal relationship to substance intoxication, withdrawal, or recent sobriety.

The first nodal point is whether the dss warrant independent clinical attention. If the answer is no, then a diagnosis of substance intoxication or withdrawal can be made (if the specific DSM-IV criteria are met). The next point of separation is whether the dss began after substance use or are etiologically related to the substance. If the answer is yes, then a diagnosis of substance-induced mood disorder with depressive features can be made. DSM-IV suggests that dss that persist for greater than 4 weeks after abstinence should not be considered as substance-induced. If the dss began prior to substance use or are not etiologically related to the substance, then the next decision is whether criteria for major depressive disorder are met. If they are, then a diagnosis of major depressive episode can be made and can be further characterized as bipolar I (if a history of mania is present) or bipolar II (if a history of hypomania is present) or as seasonal affective disorder (if those criteria are met). If a diagnosis of major depression cannot be made, then a key criterion for dysthymic disorder should be evaluated: Does the depressed mood occur more days than not for at least 2 years with other associated symptoms? If the answer is yes and other DSM IV criteria are met, then a diagnosis of dysthymic disorder can be made. Finally, if the mood develops in response to a stressor, then adjustment disorder with depressed mood should be considered, and if not, then depressive disorder not otherwise specified.

The decision tree is a helpful template, but it must be fleshed out with a more detailed consideration of the psychopathology of each diagnostic category. The criteria for substance intoxication and substance withdrawal are given in Table 1. Depressive signs and symptoms

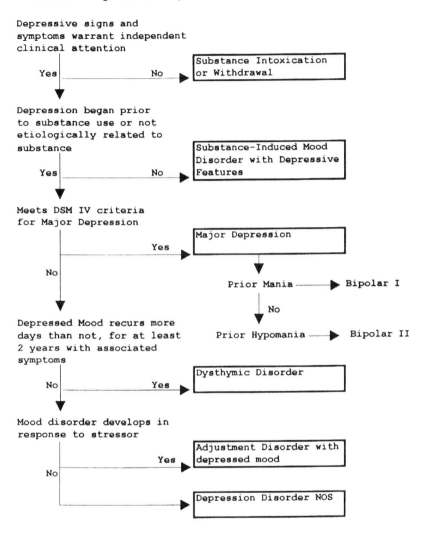

Figure 1 Decision tree distinguishing substance-related depression from primary depressive disorders. Adapted from Ref. 22, pp. 696–697.

Table 1   DSM-IV Criteria for Substance Intoxication and Withdrawal

Substance intoxication
  A. The development of a reversible substance-specific syndrome due to
     recent ingestion of (or exposure to) a substance. *Note:* Different
     substances may produce similar or identical syndromes.
  B. Clinically significant maladaptive behavioral or psychological changes
     that are due to the effect of the substance on the central nervous system
     (e.g., belligerence, mood lability, cognitive impairment, impaired
     judgment, impaired social or occupational functioning) and develop
     during or shortly after use of the substance.
  C. The symptoms are not due to a general medical condition and are not
     better accounted for by another mental disorder.

Substance withdrawal
  A. The development of a substance-specific syndrome due to the cessation
     of (or reduction in) substance use that has been heavy and prolonged.
  B. The substance-specific syndrome causes clinically significant distress
     or impairment in social, occupational, or other important areas of
     functioning.
  C. The symptoms are not due to a general medical condition and are not
     better accounted for by another mental disorder.

Source: Reprinted with permission from Ref. 22, pp. 184–185. Copyright 1994
American Psychiatric Association.

that do not require independent clinical attention are considered as part
of intoxication or withdrawal.

The more difficult distinction is between substance-induced depression and primary depressive disorders (major depression, dysthymic
disorder or adjustment disorder). Table 2 lists the criteria for substance-
induced mood disorder. Criterion C provides guidelines in distinguishing a substance-induced from a primary depressive disorder. First, onset
is an important consideration; dss that precede substance use would
favor a diagnosis of non-substance-induced mood disorder. Second,
the course of dss is relevant; dss that persist for a month or more after
substance use would also favor a non-substance-induced illness. Finally,
dss that are too severe to be related to the type or amount of substance
use would favor a diagnosis of non-substance-induced illness.

A diagnosis of a major depressive episode (MDE) (Table 3) requires
the presence of many more signs and symptoms than substance-induced

Table 2 DSM-IV Criteria for Substance-Induced Mood Disorder

A. A prominent and persistent disturbance in mood predominates in the clinical picture and is characterized by either (or both) of the following:
   (1) depressed mood or markedly diminished interest or pleasure in all, or almost all, activities
   (2) elevated, expansive, or irritable mood
B. There is evidence from the history, physical examination, or laboratory findings of either (1) or (2):
   (1) the symptoms in Criterion A developed during, or within a month of Substance Intoxication or Withdrawal
   (2) medication use is etiologically related to the disturbance
C. The disturbance is not better accounted for by a Mood Disorder that is not substance induced. Evidence that the symptoms are better accounted for by a Mood Disorder that is not substance induced might include the following: the symptoms precede the onset of the substance use (or medication use); the symptoms persist for a substantial period of time (e.g., about a month) after the cessation of acute withdrawal or severe intoxication or are substantially in excess of what would be expected given the type or amount of the substance used or the duration of use; or there is other evidence that suggests the existence of an independent non-substance-induced Mood Disorder (e.g., a history of recurrent Major Depressive Episodes).
D. The disturbance does not occur exclusively during the course of a delirium.
E. The symptoms cause clinically significant distress or impairment in social, occupational, or other important areas of functioning.

Note: This diagnosis should be made instead of a diagnosis of Substance Intoxication or Substance Withdrawal only when the mood symptoms are in excess of those usually associated with the intoxication or withdrawal syndrome and when the symptoms are sufficiently severe to warrant independent clinical attention.

Code [Specific Substance]-Induced Mood Disorder:
   (291.8 Alcohol; 292.84 Amphetamine [or Amphetamine-Like Substance]; 292.84 Cocaine; 292.84 Hallucinogen; 292.84 Inhalant; 292.84 Opioid; 292.84 Phencyclidine [or Phencyclidine-Like Substance]; 292.84 Sedative, Hypnotic, or Anxiolytic; 292.84 Other [or Unknown] Substance)

Specify type:
   With Depressive Features: if the predominant mood is depressed
   With Manic Features: if the predominant mood is elevated, euphoric, or irritable
   With Mixed Features: if symptoms of both mania and depression are present and neither predominates

Source: Reprinted with permission from Ref. 22, pp. 374–375. Copyright 1994 American Psychiatric Association.

Table 3 DSM-IV Criteria for Major Depressive Episode

A. Five (or more) of the following symptoms have been present during the same 2-week period and represent a change from previous functioning; at least one of the symptoms is either (1) depressed mood or (2) loss of interest or pleasure.
Note: Do not include symptoms that are clearly due to a general medical condition, or mood-incongruent delusions or hallucinations.
   (1) depressed mood most of the day, nearly every day, as indicated by either subjective report (e.g., feels sad or empty) or observation made by others (e.g., appears tearful). *Note:* In children and adolescents, can be irritable mood.
   (2) markedly diminished interest or pleasure in all, or almost all, activities most of the day, nearly every day (as indicated by either subjective account or observation made by others)
   (3) significant weight loss when not dieting or weight gain (e.g., a change of more than 5% of body weight in a month), or decrease or increase in appetite nearly every day. *Note:* In children, consider failure to make expected weight gains.
   (4) insomnia or hypersomnia nearly every day
   (5) psychomotor agitation or retardation nearly every day (observable by others, not merely subjective feelings of restlessness or being slowed down)
   (6) fatigue or loss of energy nearly every day
   (7) feelings of worthlessness or excessive or inappropriate guilt (which may be delusional) nearly every day (not merely self-reproach or guilt about being sick)
   (8) diminished ability to think or concentrate, or indecisiveness, nearly every day (either by subjective account or as observed by others)
   (9) recurrent thoughts of death (not just fear of dying), recurrent suicidal ideation without a specific plan, or a suicide attempt or a specific plan for committing suicide.
B. The symptoms do not meet criteria for a Mixed Episode.
C. The symptoms cause clinically significant distress or impairment in social, occupational, or other important areas of functioning.
D. The symptoms are not due to the direct physiological effects of a substance (e.g., a drug of abuse, a medication) or a general medical condition (e.g., hypothyroidism).
E. The symptoms are not better accounted for by Bereavement, i.e., after the loss of a loved one, the symptoms persist for longer than 2 months or are characterized by marked functional impairment, morbid preoccupation with worthlessness, suicidal ideation, psychotic symptoms, or psychomotor retardation.

Source: Reprinted with permission from Ref. 22, p. 327. Copyright 1994 American Psychiatric Association.

mood disorder. At least five of the nine symptoms in criterion A must be present. A study comparing organic mood syndrome, depressed types, OMS-D (which is now divided into substance-induced mood disorder and mood disorder due to a general medical condition) indicated that seven symptoms were more frequent in MDE than in OMS-D: (a) depressed mood; (b) hyposomnia; (c) decreased appetite; (d) general anxiety; (e) low self-esteem; (f) obsessions and compulsions; and (g) suicidal thoughts (21).

If a diagnosis of MDE is made, then it must be determined if this is a single (Table 4) or recurrent (Table 5) disorder and whether other specifiers apply, e.g., seasonal pattern (Table 6). In addition, if there is a past history of mania or hypomania, a diagnosis of bipolar I, depressed or bipolar II, depressed would be made. The DSM-IV criteria for mania and hypomania are given in Tables 7 and 8. It is important to note that for both mania and hypomania, the symptoms cannot be due to the direct physiological effects of substances, a general medical condition, or somatic antidepressant treatment (including medication, electroconvulsive therapy, or light therapy).

The most remarkable aspect of dysthymic disorder (Table 9) is the requirement of 2 years of depressed mood for most of the day, for more days than not. In addition, no episode of major depression can be present during the first 2 years of the disturbance.

Table 4 DSM-IV Criteria for Major Depressive Disorder, Single Episode (296.2x)

A. Presence of a single Major Depressive Episode.
B. The Major Depressive Episode is not better accounted for by Schizoaffective Disorder and is not superimposed on Schizophrenia, Schizophreniform Disorder, Delusional Disorder, or Psychotic Disorder Not Otherwise Specified.
C. There has never been a Manic Episode, a Mixed Episode, or a Hypomanic Episode. *Note:* This exclusion does not apply if all of the manic-like, mixed-like, or hypomanic-like episodes are substance or treatment induced or are due to the direct physiological effects of a general medical condition.

Source: Reprinted with permission from Ref. 22, p. 344. Copyright 1994 American Psychiatric Association.

Table 5 DSM-IV Criteria for Major Depressive Disorder, Recurrent (296.3x)

A. Presence of two or more Major Depressive Episodes.
   Note: To be considered separate episodes, there must be an interval of at least 2 consecutive months in which criteria are not met for a Major Depressive Episode.
B. The Major Depressive Episodes are not better accounted for by Schizoaffective Disorder and are not superimposed on Schizophrenia, Schizophreniform Disorder, Delusional Disorder, or Psychotic Disorder Not Otherwise Specified.
C. There has never been a Manic Episode, a Mixed Episode, or a Hypomanic Episode. *Note:* This exclusion does not apply if all of the manic-like, mixed-like, or hypomanic-like episodes are substance or treatment induced or are due to the direct physiological effects of a general medical condition.

Source: Reprinted with permission from Ref. 22, p. 345. Copyright 1994 American Psychiatric Association.

Table 6 DSM-IV Criteria for Seasonal Pattern Specifier

Specify if:
With Seasonal Pattern (can be applied to the pattern of Major Depressive Episodes in Bipolar I Disorder, Bipolar II Disorder, or Major Depressive Disorder, Recurrent)
A. There has been a regular temporal relationship between the onset of Major Depressive Episodes in Bipolar I or Bipolar II Disorder or Major Depressive Disorder, Recurrent, and a particular time of the year (e.g., regular appearance of the Major Depressive Episode in the fall or winter). *Note:* Do not include cases in which there is an obvious effect of seasonal-related psychosocial stressors (e.g., regularly being unemployed every winter).
B. Full remissions (or a change from depression to mania or hypomania) also occur at a characteristic time of the year (e.g., depression disappears in the spring).
C. In the last 2 years, two Major Depressive Episodes have occurred that demonstrate the temporal seasonal relationships defined in Criteria A and B, and no nonseasonal Major Depressive Episodes have occurred during that same period.
D. Seasonal Major Depressive Episodes (as described above) substantially outnumber the nonseasonal Major Depressive Episodes that may have occurred over the individual's lifetime.

Source: Reprinted with permission from Ref. 22, p. 390. Copyright 1994 American Psychiatric Association.

Table 7 DSM-IV Criteria for Manic Episode

A. A distinct period of abnormally and persistently elevated, expansive, or irritable mood, lasting at least 1 week (or any duration if hospitalization is necessary).
B. During the period of mood disturbance, three (or more) of the following symptoms have persisted (four if the mood is only irritable) and have been present to a significant degree:
   (1) inflated self-esteem or grandiosity
   (2) decreased need for sleep (e.g., feels rested after only 3 hours of sleep)
   (3) more talkative than usual or pressure to keep talking
   (4) flight of ideas or subjective experience that thoughts are racing
   (5) distractibility (i.e., attention too easily drawn to unimportant or irrelevant external stimuli)
   (6) increase in goal-directed activity (either socially, at work or school, or sexually) or psychomotor agitation
   (7) excessive involvement in pleasurable activities that have a high potential for painful consequences (e.g., engaging in unrestrained buying sprees, sexual indiscretions, or foolish business investments)
C. The symptoms do not meet criteria for a Mixed Episode.
D. The mood disturbance is sufficiently severe to cause marked impairment in occupational functioning or in usual social activities or relationships with others, or to necessitate hospitalization to prevent harm to self or others, or there are psychotic features.
E. The symptoms are not due to the direct physiological effects of a substance (e.g., a drug of abuse, a medication, or other treatment) or a general medical condition (e.g., hyperthyroidism).
Note: Manic-like episodes that are clearly caused by somatic antidepressant treatment (e.g., medication, electroconvulsive therapy, light therapy) should not count toward a diagnosis of Bipolar I Disorder.

Source: Reprinted with permission from Ref. 22, p. 332. Copyright 1994 American Psychiatric Association.

Now that we have completed a discussion of the criteria of the relevant DSM-IV diagnoses, we can move to a consideration of the specific substances that are correlated with these diagnoses. Table 10 summarizes the occurrence of dss in the abuse of various substances. Specifically, it indicates which substances can cause substance intoxication with depressed symptoms, substance withdrawal with depressed

Table 8 DSM-IV Criteria for Hypomanic Episode

A. A distinct period of persistently elevated, expansive, or irritable mood, lasting throughout at least 4 days, that is clearly different from the usual nondepressed mood.
B. During the period of mood disturbance, three (or more) of the following symptoms have persisted (four if the mood is only irritable) and have been present to a significant degree:
   (1) inflated self-esteem or grandiosity
   (2) decreased need for sleep (e.g., feels rested after only 3 hours of sleep)
   (3) more talkative than usual or pressure to keep talking
   (4) flight of ideas or subjective experience that thoughts are racing
   (5) distractibility (i.e., attention too easily drawn to unimportant or irrelevant external stimuli)
   (6) increase in goal-directed activity (either socially, at work or school, or sexually) or psychomotor agitation
   (7) excessive involvement in pleasurable activities that have a high potential for painful consequences (e.g., the person engages in unrestrained buying sprees, sexual indiscretions, or foolish business investments)
C. The episode is associated with an unequivocal change in functioning that is uncharacteristic of the person when not symptomatic.
D. The disturbance in mood and the change in functioning are observable by others.
E. The episode is not severe enough to cause marked impairment in social or occupational functioning, or to necessitate hospitalization, and there are no psychotic features.
F. The symptoms are not due to the direct physiological effects of a substance (e.g., a drug of abuse, a medication, or other treatment) or a general medical condition (e.g., hyperthyroidism).
Note: Hypomanic-like episodes that are clearly caused by somatic antidepressant treatment (e.g., medication, electroconvulsive therapy, light therapy) should not count toward a diagnosis of Bipolar II Disorder.

Source: Reprinted with permission from Ref. 22, p. 338. Copyright 1994 American Psychiatric Association.

Table 9 DSM-IV Criteria for Dysthymic Disorder (300.4)

A. Depressed mood for most of the day, for more days than not, as indicated either by subjective account or observation by others, for at least 2 years. *Note:* In children and adolescents, mood can be irritable and duration must be at least 1 year.

B. Presence, while depressed, of two (or more) of the following:
   (1) poor appetite or overeating
   (2) insomnia or hypersomnia
   (3) low energy or fatigue
   (4) low self-esteem
   (5) poor concentration or difficulty making decisions
   (6) feelings of hopelessness

C. During the 2-year period (1 year for children or adolescents) of the disturbance, the person has never been without the symptoms in Criteria A and B for more than 2 months at a time.

D. No Major Depressive Episode has been present during the first 2 years of the disturbance (1 year for children and adolescents); i.e., the disturbance is not better accounted for by chronic Major Depressive Disorder, or Major Depressive Disorder, In Partial Remission.
   Note: There may have been a previous Major Depressive Episode provided there was a full remission (no significant signs or symptoms for 2 months) before development of the Dysthymic Disorder. In addition, after the initial 2 years (1 year in children or adolescents) of Dysthymic Disorder, there may be superimposed episodes of Major Depressive Disorder, in which case both diagnoses may be given when the criteria are met for a Major Depressive Episode.

E. There has never been a Manic Episode, a Mixed Episode, or a Hypomanic Episode, and criteria have never been met for Cyclothymic Disorder.

F. The disturbance does not occur exclusively during the course of a chronic Psychotic Disorder, such as Schizophrenia or Delusional Disorder.

G. The symptoms are not due to the direct physiological effects of a substance (e.g., a drug of abuse, a medication) or a general medical condition (e.g., hypothyroidism).

H. The symptoms cause clinically significant distress or impairment in social, occupational, or other important areas of functioning.

Source: Reprinted with permission from Ref. 22, p. 349. Copyright 1994 American Psychiatric Association.

Table 10 Substance-Induced Depressive Disorder and Specific Classes of Substances

	Substance intox dep. symp.	Substance withdrawal dep. symp.	Substance-induced mood dis. depressive features
Alcohol	X	X	X
Amphetamine	X	X	X
Cocaine	X	X	X
Hallucinogens	X		X
Inhalants	X		X
Opioids	X		X
Phenycyclidine	X		X
Sedatives, hypnotics, anxiolytics	X	X	X

Source: Adapted from Ref. 22, p. 177. Used with permission.

symptoms, or substance-induced mood disorder with depressive features.

II. ALCOHOL AND SEDATIVES, HYPOTICS, AND ANXIOLYTICS

A number of studies indicate that alcohol intoxication produces dss in alcoholics more commonly than in nonalcoholic controls (13). Dss are also frequent during withdrawal from alcohol, but they decrease rapidly in the 4 weeks following withdrawal. A study of 191 alcoholic men indicated that 42% had significant dss as indicated by a score of 20 or greater on the Hamilton Rating Scale 1 week after abstinence (2). After 3 weeks, the figure declined to 12% and by 4 weeks to 6% (2). Other studies attest to this precipitous decline in dss (5, 6). Clearly, the bulk of patients who have undergone alcohol withdrawal will not meet criteria for MDD. Nevertheless the occurrence of MDD in abstinent alcoholics is significant. A study by Behar and Winokur of alcoholics who had maintained sobriety for at least 5 years showed that "disabling" depression occurred in 15% of the sample and the mean onset was at 35 months following sobriety (1).

In addition to MDD and dysthymia, abstinent alcoholic patients can manifest a low level of dysphoria, which Jaffe and Ciraulo have called alcoholic hypophoria (11). They found that alcoholics who have been sober for at least 6 months had more hypophoria symptoms than nonalcoholic medical inpatients.

Sedatives, hypnotics, and anxiolytics, like alcohol, can cause dss during intoxication and withdrawal and are also associated with substance-induced mood disorder. It is important to bear in mind that both depression and agitation can be so-called "paradoxical" effects of benzodiazepines (9). Withdrawal from benzodiazepines also carries the risk of dss as well as substance-induced depression (16, 18).

III. AMPHETAMINE AND COCAINE

Patients acutely intoxicated with amphetamine or cocaine can show dss, but the incidence and severity of dss increase with chronic intoxication (4, 8, 12). However, it is stimulant withdrawal that is most likely to cause dss. Gawin and Kleber reported a three-stage abstinence syndrome in chronic cocaine users (7). The first stage, which occurs within hours of abstinence, is characterized by depressed mood, agitation, fatigue, and desire to sleep. Stage 2, which occurs 1–6 days after cessation, is manifested by dysphoria, anhedonia, anxiety, and drug craving. The third and final stage, which can occur up to 10 weeks after cessation, is characterized by periodic drug craving and euthymic mood. A similar pattern exists for amphetamine withdrawal. The most severe dss occur in the 48–72 hr after discontinuation of amphetamine (12).

IV. OTHER DRUGS

Evidence exists for correlating several other drug groups with dss during substance intoxication and with substance-induced mood disorder (see Table 10). Hallucinogens, inhalants (10), opioids (13, 15, 18), and phencyclidine (3) are associated with dss during intoxication and are implicated in substance-induced mood disorder. There is some evidence for the correlation of dss with other addictions, including cannabis (4, 20) and steroids (14).

V. CONCLUSION

There are a number of strategies that a clinician can employ when confronted with addicted patients who have dss:

1. Take a careful history, which focuses on: (a) the onset of the dss in respect to the onset of the addiction; (b) whether the dss were present during a prolonged period of abstinence; (c) family history of affective disorder.
2. Do a careful mental status to determine whether the patient currently meets DSM-IV criteria for affective disorder.
3. Follow the course of the dss during the first weeks of sobriety. The majority of addicted patients who meet criteria for major depression will no longer meet criteria after 4 weeks.

Despite these and other strategies, however, the presence of dss in addicted patients will continue to be a diagnostic and therapeutic challenge. It is hoped that future research will provide clinicians with objective tests (biological, genetic, etc.) to simplify the process of differential diagnosis. Until that day, mental health professionals must continue to rely on a careful history, a skillful mental status examination, and clinical judgment.

REFERENCES

1. D. Behar and G. Winokur. Depression in the abstinent alcoholic, *Am. J. Psychiatr. 141:*1106–1107 (1984).
2. S. A. Brown and M. A. Schuckikt. Changes in depression among abstinent alcoholics, *J. Stud. Alcohol 49:*412–417 (1988).
3. G. Caracci, P. Mignoni, and S. Mukherjee. Phencyclidine abuse and depression, *Psychosomatics 24:*932–933 (1983).
4. C. Ciolino. Substance abuse and mood disorders, *Dual Diagnosis in Substance Abuse* (M. S. Gold and A. E. Slaby, eds.), Marcel Dekker, New York, 1991, pp. 105–115.
5. D. Clark, R. F. D. Gibbons, M. G. Gaviland et al., Assessing the severity of depressive states in recently detoxified alcoholics, *J. Stud. Alcohol 54:*107–114 (1993).
6. K. M. Davidson. Diagnosis of depression in alcohol dependence: changes in prevalence with drinking status, *Br. J. Psychiatr. 166:*199–204 (1995).

7. F. H. Gawin and H. D. Kleber. Abstinence symptomatology and psychiatric diagnosis in cocaine abusers: clinical observations, *Arch. Gen. Psychiatr. 43:*107–113 (1986).

8. F. H. Gawin and E. H. Ellinwood. Cocaine and other stimulants: actions, abuse, and treatment, *N. Engl. J. Med. 318:*1173–1182 (1988).

9. R. C. Hall and S. Zisook. Paradoxical reactions to benzodiazepines, *Br. J. Clin. Pharmacol. 11:*995–1045 (1981).

10. A. M. Jacobs and A. Hamnid-Ghodse. Depression in solvent abusers, *Soc. Sci. Med. 24:*863–866 (1987).

11. J. H. Jaffe and D. A. Ciraulo. Alcoholism and depression, *Psychopathology and Addictive Disorders* (R. E. Meyer, ed.), Guilford Press, New York, 1985, pp. 293–320.

12. J. Jaffe. Drug addiction and drug use, *The Pharmacological Basis of Therapeutics,* 8th ed. (A. G. Gilman, T. W. Rall, A. S. Nies et al., eds.) Pergamon Press, New York, 1990.

13. H. R. Kranzler and N. R. Liebowitz. Anxiety and depression in substance abuse: clinical implication. *Med. Clin. North Am. 72*(4):867–885 (1988).

14. D. A. Malone and R. J. Dimeff. The use of fluxoetine in depression associated with anabolic steroid withdrawal: a case series. *J. Clin. Psychiatr. 53:*130–132 (1992).

15. W. R. Martin, C. A. Haertzen and B. B. Hewett. Psychopathology and pathophysiology of narcotic addicts, alcoholics and drug abusers, *Psychopharmacology: A Generation of Progress.* (M. A. Lipton, A. DiMascio, and K. F. Killam, eds.). Raven Press, New York, 1978.

16. D. Olajide and M. Lader. Depression following withdrawal from long-term benzodiazepine use. A report of four cases. *Psychol. Med. 14:* 937 (1984).

17. D. A. Regier, M. E. Farmer, D. S. Rae, et al. Comorbidity of mental disorders with alcohol and drug abuse. *JAMA 264:*2511–2518 (1990).

18. J. A. Renner and D. A. Ciraulo. Substance abuse and depression. *Psychiatr. Ann. 24:*532–539 (1994).

19. H. E. Ross, F. B. Glaser, and T. Germanson. The prevalence of psychiatric disorders in patients with alcohol and other drug problems. *Arch. Gen. Psychiatr. 45:*1023–1031 (1988).

20. H. Thomas. Psychiatric symptoms in cannabis users, *Br. J. Psychiatr. 163:*141–149 (1993).

21. U.R. Cornelius, H. Fabrega, J. Mezzick, et al. Characterizing organic mood syndrome, depressed type, *Compr. Psychiatry 34:*432–440 (1993).

22. DSM–IV, Diagnostic and Statistical Manual of Mental Disorders, ed. 4. American Psychiatric Association, Washington, D.C., 1994.

3

Treatment for Adjustment Disorder with Depressed Mood

Willa Bernhard
Cornell University Medical College, New York, New York

I. INTRODUCTION

There has been a considerable amount of information about the treatment of adjustment disorder and addiction, and on short-term therapies for depression, but there has been no information on an integrative approach for the treatment of a patient in recovery who is suffering from an adjustment disorder with depressed mood.

To review, according to DSM-IV, adjustment disorders are characterized by a maladaptive response or reaction to an identifiable psychosocial stressor or stressors. The emotional or behavioral symptoms must have occurred within 3 months of the onset of the stressor(s). The symptoms that exceed ''normal or expected'' reactions include impairment of significant social, interpersonal, or work functions. The predominant features of an adjustment disorder with depressed mood are symptoms such as depressed mood, tearfulness, or feelings of hopelessness. Stressors may be recurrent or continuous (1).

The patient recovering from addiction is at particular risk for an adjustment disorder. Depression of varying degrees of severity is a

27

common experience during all phases of recovery. In a study at Stanford Alcohol Clinic at Stanford University, 89.6% of respondents reported experiencing periods of depression after becoming abstinent (2). Others who work with patients in recovery report similar findings.

The individual in recovery from addiction is contending with multiple psychosocial stressors, including problems in personal, familial, and occupational functioning, grief at the loss of the addictive substance, the separation from friends and companions, shame, guilt, the loss of a way of life, and a familiar sense of one's identity (2). The recovering addict's life is often in disarray at a time when the habitual way of reducing stress, the use of alcohol, drugs, or other addictive behaviors, is no longer available, and when the defenses that protected the addict from the reality of his actions and his situation, mainly denial and rationalization, no longer protect him.

Clinical studies indicate that most addicts have suffered emotional and psychological deprivation during their childhood and, as a result, lack the problem-solving and coping skills needed to meet the challenges necessary for a satisfactory adjustment to life.

Many patients in recovery were themselves the children of addicted parents. Beletsis and Brown, in studies of this population, characterize the homes in which children of alcoholics grow up as being beset by chaos, inconsistency, unclear roles, arbitrariness, changing limits, repetitious and illogical arguments, and perhaps violence and incest (3). ''Because of the nature of the environment, members of the family expend enormous amounts of energy just to cope with their external world. So much effort goes into denial and coping with the chaotic reality that there is little energy left for internal development'' (4). Many addicts, particularly women, have been sexually abused during childhood or adolescence.

Rohsenow, Corbett, and Devine report that up to 75% of women and 16% of men were sexually abused as youths. Psychosis or other serious mental illness is common among members of an addict's family. Studies indicate a correlation between severe difficulties in early mothering experiences, object loss during childhood or adolescence, and addiction (5). Much evidence supports the view that negative developmental experiences play a significant role in adult adjustment.

A psychodynamic interpretation of the psychopathology of alcohol addiction is that a significant degree of deprivation during early childhood can produce adults with greater than usual conflicts because of their excessive dependency needs. Zimberg (6) writes,

> Childhood rejection, overprotection, or premature responsibility leads to an unconscious need for nurturance which cannot be met in reality and results in rejection. The rejection leads to anxiety, which in turn leads to the development of a number of defense mechanisms, particularly denial, and a compensatory need for grandiosity. The grandiosity causes such individuals to try harder and results in inevitable failure. The failures lead to more depression, anger and guilt. These unpleasant affects can be reduced by alcohol, at least for a time, and lead to pharmacologically induced feelings of power and omnipotence, thus reinforcing the denial and reactive grandiosity.

The perspective on substance use and abuse and other addictive behaviors derived from stress coping theory provides a useful and practical theoretical and treatment orientation for patients in recovery who are suffering from adjustment disorders. Stress coping theory (SCT) postulates that substance use and abuse represents a habitual maladaptive coping response to temporarily decrease life stresses. According to this theoretical framework, substance abuse is an adaptive process involving cognitive, social learning mechanisms. Addiction is an extreme, dysfunctional, and harmful way of dealing with life's problems, but it is an essential part of the addict's ecology and can't be relinquished until better and healthier ways of coping with stress have been learned.

This defective psychosocial learning process damages the person's ability to cope and derive stable sources of gratification. The addict's psychosocial skills deficits must be addressed and remedied before the individual can give up substance use as the way to cope with life's stresses and strains. This compensatory model places emphasis on training in social skills and acquiring social competencies (7).

II. TREATMENT CONSIDERATIONS

Generally speaking, the treatment of an adjustment disorder is oriented toward improving the patient's level of adaptation. This is accomplished by using environmental manipulation to remove the stressor(s) and psychotherapy to explore the patient's attitude and, hopefully, to change his perspective (8).

The literature on the treatment of an adjustment disorder often presupposes that the patient had a satisfactory homeostasis before becoming overwhelmed by psychosocial stressors, and the immediate goal is to help the patient get back what has been lost.

When developing a treatment plan for patients recovering from addiction, it is necessary to recognize their need to find, probably for the first time, an addiction-free homeostasis.

With patients in recovery, treatment for an adjustment disorder with depressed mood must be geared to the individual's needs at a particular point in the recovery continuum. Abstinence in early recovery is the middle or beginning of a larger process. The patient's needs will be different at various stages of recovery. In early recovery, the major focus in the patient's life is to remain abstinent. The patient needs constant behavioral, cognitive, and object reminders that provide external support. This is a time of extreme stress. The loss of protective and familiar defenses leaves the patient newly aware of his circumstances, including damages from the past and the flood of feelings that were medicated by the substance or kept from awareness by protective defenses.

Family, friends, and business associates see these patients as cured and expect them to function in a mentally healthy manner. The patient, without the substance and the old way of life, is very dependent and needs to rely on external structure and support until a new identity emerges. The external structure provides a safe place for developing the necessary adaptive behavioral, cognitive, problem-solving, and interpersonal skills.

The therapy for patients recovering from an addiction, who are suffering from an adjustment disorder with depressed mood, must be designed to help them overcome the depression as quickly as possible. There are psychodynamic, cognitive, behavioral, and interpersonally oriented, brief, focused treatment models that can be effective for many depressed patients. There will be some patients who will not respond to nonpharmacological treatment alone and will need to combine antidepressant medication with therapy.

Before therapy begins, an evaluation should be made as to whether an antidepressant is indicated. If a decision is made to treat the patient without medication, and if the depression does not remit, it is important to reevaluate the earlier decision.

If the patient is not improving, a diagnosis of a major depressive disorder should be considered. Chapter 4, on the treatment of a major depressive disorder, outlines the therapeutic use of antidepressant medication.

Viewing the depression as part of a larger problem, the treatment plan might also include an educational component, family sessions, and group therapy. A support group, such as Alcoholics Anonymous (AA), often plays a very important part in the patient's recovery. Crisis intervention therapy has been recommended by the Task Force Report of the American Psychiatric Association as a practical treatment option for adjustment disorders (8). It is brief, focused, and goal directed; the goal is to resolve the crisis that occurs when a person is overwhelmed by stress. Crisis intervention therapy synthesizes aspects from psychiatry, psychology, social work, public health, and sociology.

One of its advantages is that it can be used by therapists from various disciplines who can adapt their particular training and orientation to the core of therapeutic concepts that are basic to crisis intervention theory.

The crisis intervention model is a treatment format that can embrace and integrate different therapeutic modalities; the format can be individualized to meet the patient's needs. Crisis intervention treatment sets parameters; within the parameters, the therapist is free to use the treatment modalities best suited to the patient's needs and the therapist's orientation. Swanson and Carbon have compiled the therapeutic concepts that are basic to crisis intervention theory (9).

1. Crises are normal life experiences and do not represent illness or pathology. An emotional crisis reflects a realistic struggle in which the individual works to maintain a state of equilibrium between himself and his surroundings (10).
2. The stress that brings on the crisis may be either an internal or an external event (11). It may occur as a single catastrophic event or as a series of milder happenings that may have a cumulative effect (12).
3. The severity of the crisis is not directly related to the severity of the stressor; it is a function, rather, of the individual's perception of the event (13).

4. There may be a link between the individual's current situation and past conflicts. This connection is experienced emotionally by the patient (14).
5. Emotional crises are self-limiting events. The period of acute disorganization is usually resolved within 4 to 6 weeks, with either adaptive or maladaptive results (15).
6. Individuals in a state of crisis have weakened defenses. This increased vulnerability makes them more amenable to help (16). A minimal effort at this time can have maximal effect (13).
7. Adaptive crisis resolution offers a triple opportunity, first to master the present situation, second, to rework some past conflicts, and third, to learn better ways to deal with crises in the future (10).
8. Adaptive crisis resolution is not determined by past experiences or character structure, but by processes occurring in the present (17).
9. An inherent component of every crisis is an actual or anticipated loss experienced by the individual. Reconciling this loss is part of the crisis resolution process (18, 19).
10. With adaptive crisis resolution, new ego sets emerge as new coping and problem-solving skills are developed that will help the individual in the future (20).

Crisis intervention is a time-limited therapy with well-defined goals. The therapist is supportive; a positive patient-therapist relationship is essential, but the emphasis remains on helping the patient help himself. Support systems drawn from family, friends, and community are enlisted as needed. Treatment is divided into four phases: (i) an assessment of the current situation; (ii) an initial formulation of treatment goals; (iii) implementing the treatment strategies designed to help the patient develop the skills necessary to resolve the crisis; (iv) resolution of the crisis (9).

The assessment phase and the initial formulation of treatment goals are usually accomplished in the first session. The assessment should include an estimation of the patient's present situation, the problem that seems most relevant to the patient's depression, what coping mechanisms the patient is using, and an evaluation of how they are working.

It is important to evaluate the patient's strengths so they can be mobilized in the treatment. Because all crises involve real or imagined loss, it is important to determine how the loss affects the immediate problem.

An assessment should be made of the patient's family, social, and community support systems. It is also important in the first session to determine whether the patient is suicidal or a threat to others.

The information gathered during the assessment should inform the treatment goals. The goals should be specific and attainable in brief treatment. Treatment must address what the patient feels are his significant problems and needs. The patient should understand that when the treatment goals have been reached, the crisis intervention therapy will end.

One or more therapeutic modalities might be used in the implementation phase of treatment. The therapist uses the data collected to decide what dysfunctional themes, behaviors, and cognitions need to be addressed in the therapy sessions. It is important for the therapist and patient to agree on treatment goals.

Problem-solving therapy, cognitive therapy, and interpersonal therapy, all focused, brief treatment modalities presented in Chapters 9, 10, and 11 can be used to give patients necessary cognitive, behavioral, and interpersonal skills.

It is recommended in crisis intervention therapy that family members be brought into the treatment for at least one session because of the importance of family and social supports. Much damage can be done by the family that sabotages treatment because they are discouraged or lack understanding of the process. Family treatment for one or more sessions is particularly important when the patient is recovering from addiction because both the addiction and the recovery process greatly affect the members and dynamics of the family. Insight-oriented, uncovering, psychodynamic psychotherapy can be helpful to patients in later stages of recovery. It is not recommended for those in early recovery when the newly abstinent patient is vulnerable, dependent, and in need of support and day-to-day problem-solving and coping skills.

The therapist should have knowledge of community resources that may be available to the patient. Help in obtaining housing, a referral for medical help, or information about a support group can be important adjuncts to therapy.

When a patient is in a support group such as AA, the therapy and the support group should reinforce each other because both fill important roles in the patient's rehabilitation and mental health recovery.

The last phase of treatment is termination. As this phase nears, the patient should be aware that treatment is drawing to a close because an ongoing part of therapy has been an assessment of the patient's progress in meeting goals. Treatment should draw to a close when the depression has abated and the patient feels better. Feelings about termination should be discussed in the last few sessions.

Loss and separation are problems for many if not most people. Because feelings about loss and separation precipitated the crisis, the patient has much to gain by being able to express to the therapist any feelings about ending the relationship. The patient may also learn that feeling a sense of loss when relationships end is natural and a part of the experience of living.

During this last stage, the patient and the therapist should review the course of the therapy and identify the patient's newly acquired coping and problem-solving skills. If the patient and the therapist share a sense of enthusiasm about the work they have done together, as well as optimism about the future, the patient is more likely to feel positive about what lies ahead.

It is important to bring the crisis therapy to an end so the patient can begin the next phase with a sense of success about the completed treatment.

Before the crisis therapy ends, both patient and therapist should assess whether further treatment is needed. Therapy should end with the understanding that if help is needed in the future, the therapist can be contacted.

In summary, treatment modalities that can be used in crisis intervention with this population include interpersonal psychotherapy, cognitive therapy, and problem-solving therapy. Chapters 9, 10, and 11 serve as excellent guides for modalities that have proved successful in treating depression. Other brief treatment interventions that can be used include behavior therapy, family treatment, and group therapy. Individual psychodynamic psychotherapy can be a very helpful modality that should be reserved for a later stage in the recovery process.

REFERENCES

1. R. D. Coddington, Adjustment disorder: Introduction, *A Task Force Report of the American Psychiatric Association,* Vol. 3, Washington, D.C., 1989, pp. 1046–1049.

2. S. Brown, *Treating the Alcoholic: A Developmental Model of Recovery,* John Wiley and Sons, 1985, p. 53.

3. S. Beletsis and S. Brown, A developmental framework for understanding the children of alcoholics. Focus on women, *Journal of Health and the Addictions 2:*1–32 (1981).

4. T. Cermak and S. Brown, Interactional group psychotherapy with the children of alcoholics, *Int. J. Group Psychother. 32(3):*375–789 (1982).

5. D. J. Rohsenow, R. Corbett and E. Devine, Molested as children: A hidden contribution to substance abuse, *Journal of Abuse Treatment 5:*13–18 (1988).

6. S. Zimberg, Principles of alcoholism psychotherapy, *Practical Approaches to Alcoholism Psychotherapy* (S. Zimberg, J. Wallace, and S. Blume, eds.) Plenum Press, New York, 1978, pp. 3.–17.

7. R. C. Hawkins, Substance abuse and stress coping resources: A life contextual clinical viewpoint, *The Chemically Dependent: Phases of Treatment and Recovery* (Barbara C. Wallace, ed.), Brunner/Mazel, New York, 1992.

8. J. Hutzler, Adjustment disorders in adulthood and old age, *A Task Force Report of the American Psychiatric Association,* Vol. 3, Washington, D.C. 1989, pp. 2504–2510.

9. W. C. Swanson and J. B. Carbon, Crisis intervention, theory and technique. Treatment of Psychiatric Disorders, *A Task Force Report of the American Psychiatric Association,* Vol. 3, Washington, D.C. 1989, pp. 2520–2531.

10. G. Caplan, *Principles of Preventive Psychotherapy,* Basic Books, New York, 1964,

11. E. H. Erikson, *Childhood and Society,* Norton, New York, 1950.

12. I. Korner, Crisis reduction and the psychological consultant, *Crisis Intervention* (G. Spector and W. Claiborn, eds.), Behavioral Publications, New York, (1973).

13. L. Rapoport, The state of crisis: Some theoretical considerations, *Social Service Review 36:*211–217 (1962).
14. D. Hoffman and M. Remmel, Uncovering the precipitant in crisis intervention, *Soc. Casework 56:*259 (1975).
15. B. Bloom, *Community Mental Health: A General Introduction,* Brooks/ Cole, Monterey, 1977
16. S. Schwartz, A review of crisis intervention programs, *Psychiatric Quarterly 45:*498–508 (1971).
17. L. Paul, Crisis intervention, *Mental Hygiene 50:*141–145 (1966).
18. J. Hitchcock, Crisis intervention: The pebble in the pool, *American J. of Nursing 73:*1388–1390 (1973).
19. M. Strickler, B. LaSor, The concept of loss in crisis intervention, *Mental Hygiene 54:*301–305 (1970).
20. N. Golan, *Treatment in Crisis Situations,* Free Press, New York, 1978.
21. R. H. Moos, J. Finney and R. Cronkite, *Alcoholism Treatment, Context, Process and Outcome,* Oxford University Press, New York, 1990.
22. J. Noshpitz, *Individual Psychotherapy in Adjustment Disorders, Stresses and the Adjustment Disorders* (J. Noshphitz and R. Dean Coddington, eds.), John Wiley and Sons, New York, 1990.
23. M. J. Horowitz, Brief dynamic psychotherapy, *A Task Force Report of the American Psychiatric Association,* Vol. 3, Washington, D.C., 1989, pp. 2548–2556.
24. E. M. Beal, Family therapy, *A Task Force Report of the American Psychiatric Association,* Vol. 3, Washington, D.C., 1989, pp. 2566–2578.
25. L. D. Bormon, Self help and mutual aid groups for adults, *A Task Force Report of the American Psychiatric Association,* Vol. 3, Washington, D.C., pp. 2596–2607.

4

Treatment for Major Depressive Disorder

Timothy I. Mueller

Brown University School of Medicine and Butler Hospital,
Providence, Rhode Island

I. INTRODUCTION

A treatise on the treatment of major depressive disorder in people who are in early recovery from chemical dependency presumes that the difficult questions addressed in earlier chapters of this book have been answered. It is a challenge to establish the diagnosis of major depressive disorder in the context of regular use of psychoactive chemicals. Many of these drugs have direct depressive effects, have depressive symptoms as sequellae of withdrawal states, and are associated with adverse psychosocial consequences that can trigger both depression and drug use (1–10). Not only is there this interaction of psychoactive drugs and mood, but the co-occurrence of dependence and abuse syndromes and major depressive disorder may also represent the co-occurrence of two common and chronic disorders. There are circumstances in which the diagnosis of major depressive disorder in the presence of a psychoactive substance use disorder is best viewed as provisional. This recognizes the importance of time as a diagnostic tool.

In addition to the challenge of establishing the diagnosis, treatment must overcome other hurdles that have characterized the care of the dually diagnosed. The long-standing stereotypes of the psychiatric vs the twelve-step approaches to treatment in this population represent seemingly irreconcilable positions (11). Fortunately this is evolving toward resolution. On one hand, the emergence of the American Society of Addiction Medicine (ASAM) and the American Academy of Psychiatrists in Alcoholism and Addictions (aaPaa) represents the development of special chemical dependency expertise among physicians. On the other hand, Alcoholics Anonymous' official acknowledgment of the value of psychiatric medications represents an acceptance of the place for judicious pharmacotherapy (12). Despite these developments, I continue to hear my colleagues in psychiatry regularly report that their patients' use of abusive drugs is secondary to their depression or anxiety or some other symptom complex, and that psychotherapy aimed at their ''underlying disorder'' will cure them. I also hear my patients report the need to conceal their use of psychiatric medications from their AA friends in order to avoid the rejection they feel they would endure for using a ''mind-altering chemical.'' This is not an easy area for us or for our patients.

II. EPIDEMIOLOGY

There have been two major approaches to quantifying the number of people with the overlap of major depressive disorder and psychoactive substance abuse and dependence—community-based and clinical population-based epidemiological studies. Clinical epidemiology has been characterized by the nearly universal use of dimensional measures of depressive syndromes and the use of scale score cut-offs to define depression (13). This approach may overestimate the occurrence of major depressive disorder and has resulted in the dramatic statement that between 3%–98% of people in alcohol treatment have depression (14). If in adopting a dimensional approach to the depression assessment, we look at people who have significantly elevated scores, and if we then use this as an approximation for clinically significant depression, it appears that approximately 20%–40% of people with alcohol or drug dependencies have significant depressive symptoms (15–17).

Community-based samples provide a somewhat different view. Typically, these studies look at the lifetime prevalence of disorders and generally use interview tools that arrive at categorical diagnoses. The results are more generalizable to a non–treatment-seeking population and support the high co-occurrence of the two disorders (18–20). The Epidemiologic Catchment Area (ECA) study of over 20,000 people in five communities in the United States has demonstrated that approximately 27% of people with major depressive disorder have a lifetime diagnosis of psychoactive substance abuse or dependence. Conversely, 12% of the people with psychoactive substance abuse or dependence have a lifetime diagnosis of major depressive disorder. Both of these rates of co-occurrence exceed the general community lifetime prevalence of 14% for psychoactive substance abuse and dependence, and 6% for major depressive disorder.

Establishing the link between the two disorders is useful for outlining the scope of the problem and guiding public policy decisions for prioritizing health care resources. This exercise, however, has its limitations in that it does not necessarily provide an explanation for the link, nor does it offer data for successful treatment applications. The high co-occurrence of psychoactive substance dependence and abuse and psychiatric disorders, especially major depressive disorder, has generated many explanatory models, including the self-medication hypothesis (21), the depression spectrum disorder (22), kindling (23, 24), the tridimensional personality disorder (25), and genetic hypotheses (26–28). It has also led to extensive research in the area of treatment applications (29). It is this latter area that is the subject of this chapter.

III. DIAGNOSTIC CONSIDERATIONS:

The challenge of establishing the diagnosis of major depressive disorder and psychoactive substance abuse and dependence is described in Chapter 3. There is perfect overlap between the symptoms of major depressive disorder and the organic affective symptoms of psychoactive substance intoxication and withdrawal. Nothing phenomenologically distinguishes these symptoms (30). In an attempt to clarify the confusion the field has largely attempted to create hierarchies of diagnosis. The Diagnostic and Statistical Manual (DSM-III-R) and its companion diagnostic instrument, the Structured Clinical Interview for DSM-III-R (SCID), exclude symptoms of major depressive disorder in the presence of psychoactive drug use (Table 4–1). This serves to provide clarity in applying diagnostic criteria, but at the expense of discarding criteria for major depressive disorder in people who are unable to maintain periods of abstinence.

The primary and secondary classification is another attempt at establishing clarity. Unfortunately, there is a lack of uniformity in definitions for primary or secondary disorders. The definitions range from strictly chronological (which one comes first), to which is most dominant (which one causes the most trouble), to which the patient identifies as the most important. Despite proclamations in the literature that the primary and secondary distinction has clinical utility, i.e., the primary disorder more consistently characterizes the course (11, 31–33), there is little empiric evidence that primary and secondary diagnostic categories distinguish course or clinical outcome characteristics in people with clear major depressive disorder (34–36). In the absence of clear biological markers for major depressive disorder and psychoactive substance abuse and dependence, we must rely on the phenomenology. Current

Table 1   Major Depressive Disorder—DSM-III-R Diagnostic Criteria*

A. At least five of the following symptoms have been present for 2 weeks with at least one symptom from items 1 or 2.
  1. Depressed mood
  2. Anhedonia—markedly diminished interest or pleasure in life activities
  3. Significant weight loss or gain, or significant appetite increase or decrease
  4. Insomnia or hypersomnia
  5. Psychomotor retardation or agitation
  6. Anergy—loss of energy
  7. Worthlessness or excessive guilt
  8. Loss of concentration
  9. Recurrent thoughts of death or suicide
B. There is no known organic cause for the mood state.
C. Delusions or hallucinations, if present, occur in the presence of the mood disturbance.

---

*Adapted from American Psychiatric Association, 1987.

wisdom suggests that major depressive disorder can be accurately diagnosed if it occurs chronologically before psychoactive substance abuse or dependence, or occurs during periods of abstinence. In addition, because most people's use of psychoactive drugs waxes and wanes over time, chronic and persistent symptoms of major depressive disorder likely represent co-occurring disorders (37). Requiring 4 weeks of persistent symptoms in the presence of documented abstinence is diagnostically conservative but may be too high a threshold. The danger of less restrictive criteria lies in overdiagnosis and subsequent unnecessary treatment of what may not actually be major depressive disorder. Overtreatment is rarely the problem as there is ample evidence demonstrating inadequate treatment of major depressive disorder alone or in combination with alcoholism (38, 39). Ultimately, the decision to treat becomes a risk/benefits analysis. Because there is a broad choice of possible treatments, it is often the case that the risks of treatment are not substantial compared to the potential benefits.

The presence or absence of major depressive disorder in recovery has clinical meaning in addition to the treatment implications. Co-occurring psychoactive substance abuse and dependence and depression are associated with increased rates of suicide (40). The presence of psychopathology predicts poor alcohol and drug treatment outcomes (41–44). The presence of persistent alcoholism or a diagnosis of alcoholism predicts poor outcomes for major depressive disorder (45, 46). Also, the knowledge is clinically relevant in advising patients about the time course of their disorders and in collaborating with them on treatment decisions.

IV. TREATMENT

Assuming we have settled the issues of diagnosis (see Chapter 2) and are receptive to any effective treatment modality for people who are in recovery from chemical dependency and also have major depressive disorder, we can tackle the challenges of therapy. Fortunately, there are many options for treatment of this disorder in people in early recovery from chemical dependency (47, 48). In fact, there are few contraindications to the application of any of the standard treatments for major depressive disorder. Some treatments may have unique applicability in this population. Additionally, sobriety-focused treatments may be useful in the treatment of major depressive disorder beyond what they provide by simply reinforcing abstinence. The recently published practice guidelines for major depressive disorder are an excellent guide (49).

An important first step to the diagnosis of major depressive disorder is ruling out medical causes. Standard texts offer excellent advice in this regard (50). However, there are sequellae of psychoactive substance abuse that increase the likelihood of certain medical disorders (Table 4–2). Having ruled out or treated the medical causes of major depressive disorder, we are left with several broad categories for treatment options, including abstinence, somatic treatment, nonsomatic treatment (i.e. psychotherapy), and unconventional treatments.

A. Abstinence

It is not possible to overemphasize the importance of abstinence in the treatment of major depressive disorder. In the short run, most depressive syndromes resolve with abstinence (51, 52, 53, 54). In the long run, in people with confidentially diagnosed major depressive disorder and alcoholism, the persistence of active alcoholism predicts poor outcomes. A 10-year prospective follow-up study using subjects who initially presented for treatment of affective syndromes demonstrated that the persistence of evidence of active alcoholism predicted half the likelihood of improvement in major depressive disorder compared with

Table 2 Differential Diagnostic Considerations—Major Depressive Disorder and Psychoactive Substance Abuse and Dependence

Head injury—especially closed head injury
Epilepsy—often secondary to head injury, especially temporal lobe epilepsy
Central nervous system tumors metastatic from primary sources, i.e., head and neck, pulmonary, gastrointestinal
HIV disease from intravenous drug use and high-risk sexual acts
Embolic and infectious strokes from intravenous drug use
Diabetes mellitus secondary to alcoholic pancreatis
Metabolic encephalopathy secondary to liver failure
Nutritional deficiencies—B12, folate, thiamine

depressive subjects also comorbid for alcoholism who had no evidence of active alcoholism (46). Whether this effect is a nonspecific effect of abstinence or some antidepressant activity of abstinence-based treatment is an interesting question. In the absence of an answer, it is clear that abstinence increases the likelihood of improvement from major depressive disorder.

B. Somatic Treatments

Most of the somatic treatments for major depressive disorder have been tried as specific treatments to support abstinence independent of the presence of major depressive disorder. This is not the focus of this chapter; however secondary analyses of depressed vs nondepressed subjects in many of these studies are the source of data to address this issue. The literature provides little support for the use of antidepressive pharmacotherapy for abstinence itself in the absence of major depressive disorder. Selective serotonergic reuptake inhibitors (SSRIs) may be an exception (Table 4–3).

1. Tricyclic Antidepressants

Tricyclic antidepressants (TCA) are a valuable and "old" treatment for major depressive disorder (55). There is extensive research on the use of TCAs in alcoholic populations, with a smaller body of work in

Table 3 Pharmacotherapeutic Choices for the Treatment of Major Depressive Disorder

Tricyclic Antidepressants	*Selective Serotonergic*
Amitriptyline (Elavil and others)	*Reuptake Inhibitors*
Imipramine (Tofranil and others)	Fluoxetine (Prozac)
Desipramine (Norpramin and others)	Sertraline (Zoloft)
Nortriptyline (Pamelor and others)	Paroxetine (Paxil)
Doxepin (Sinequan and others)	*Miscellaneous Agents*
Clomipramine (Anafranil)	Bupropion (Wellbutrin)
Monoamine Oxidase Inhibitors	Trazodone (Desyrel)
Tranylcypromine (Parnate)	Carbamazepine (Tegretol)
Phenelzine (Nardil)	
Isocarboxazid (Marplan)	

drug populations (9, 56–62). It does not appear that TCAs have much clinical activity in the support of sobriety. They may, however, be helpful in that group of alcohol and drug abusers who have depressive symptoms. Recent systematic work on the application of TCAs in alcoholics provides additional support for this finding. Mason's report of a placebo-controlled double-blind study of desipramine in depressed alcoholics with serum drug level monitoring showed that desipramine was associated with an improvement in depression but no difference in measures of sobriety (63). Nunes demonstrated similar results with an open trial of imipramine in 60 depressed alcoholics. In addition, there were improvements in drinking behavior (64).

However, it is useful to exercise some caution in the application of these therapeutic agents. Most studies evaluating the effectiveness of TCAs have not monitored serum levels of tricyclic antidepressants. There is evidence that alcohol decreases TCA levels, suggesting that they need to be followed to accurately gauge drug efficacy (65). There is also the potential of increased sedative interaction when combining TCAs and sedative drugs of abuse. Tricyclic antidepressants lower the seizure threshold, which has the potential to complicate seizures seen in alcohol or barbiturate withdrawal and may increase the likelihood of seizures during acute cocaine intoxication. The anticholinergic effect of most TCAs may aggravate the memory deficits common in alcohol and sedative dependence. The antihistamine effects of the TCAs lead to marked mucous membrane dryness in sensitive individuals. This may increase the thickness of respiratory secretions, with the attendant risk of aggravating respiratory disorders. This population is already at increased risk for chronic respiratory disorders secondary to comorbid tobacco use and the respiratory trauma that can occur in states of deep sedation.

2. Monoamine Oxidase Inhibitors

There is scant empirical work on the use of monoamine oxidase inhibitors (MAOI) for major depressive disorder in recovery. One study of seven subjects provides negative evidence for their utility (66). The main difficulty in the application of MAOIs lies in the toxicity that occurs with dietary indiscretion of tyramine-containing foods and wines and the abusive use of meperidine and central nervous system stimulants (cocaine, amphetamines). The interaction of these drugs with MAOIs can lead to sympathomimetic crises with hypertension and an increased risk of cerebral vascular strokes. Despite my clinical impression that many alcoholics display a depressive syndrome similar to atypical depression (i.e., major depression with hypersomnia, increased appetite, and rejection sensitivity), and that MAOIs may be uniquely helpful in this disorder (67–69), it appears best to avoid their use or to use them with extreme caution.

3. Lithium

There is a large body of research on the use of lithium as an adjunct to sobriety (70–73). Early studies appeared to support the utility of lithium in maintaining sobriety; however, much of this work suffered from methodological flaws. Additionally, when broadly applied in clinical populations, lithium had no apparent value in maintaining abstinence. The study by Dorus et al. of 457 male veteran alcoholics demonstrated that lithium had no effect on sobriety in this population whether or not affective symptoms were present (74). However, it proved to be safe and to show some efficacy in decreasing symptoms of depression as measured by the Beck Depression Inventory. Lithium is more typically used as the primary treatment in bipolar disorder or as an adjunct to antidepressants in treatment-resistant major depressive disorder (75). The use of lithium presents few contraindications in early recovery. In actively drinking populations, the combined diuretic effect of alcohol (suppression of antidiuretic hormone) and lithium (associated with a syndrome of inappropriate antidiuretic hormone suppression) may lead to excess free-water loss and states of dehydration.

4. Selective Serotonergic Reuptake Inhibitors

Animal models demonstrate that the SSRI lead to a decrease in alcohol intake. This is hypothesized to be due primarily to the involvement of the serotonergic transmitter systems in the appetitive neuronal pathways (76–78). These findings have led to an enthusiastic search for the appropriate clinical use of these medications in humans. The evidence is preliminary and mixed for alcoholism. Fluoxetine compared with placebo is associated with a clinically meaningful decrease in alcohol intake in nonalcoholic problem drinkers. This difference was a statistically nonsignificant trend and was not mediated through changes in measures of depression (79). Certainly, SSRIs are effective medications in the treatment of major depressive disorder (80). If the specific abstinence supporting effects hold up to the test of further scientific inquiry, they may be the treatment of choice in this population with both diagnoses.

In addition, the SSRIs have advantages over other antidepressant medications. They are currently experiencing a vogue of popular interest (81). They have minimal side effects when compared with older tricyclic antidepressants. There is little pharmacological interaction with most other medications or drugs of abuse. As with other antidepressants, they have the potential to lower the seizure threshold in people at risk of convulsive disorders; however, this risk appears to be lower for SSRIs than for other antidepressants (80).

5. *Miscellaneous*

Although other newer pharmacological agents such as buproprion may be useful, they have no specific indications in this population. Buproprion has the potential of being more epileptogenic than other antidepressants, although this appears to be quite low when it is used within the recommended range. Trazodone is an antidepressant positioned between the sedating TCAs and the SSRIs in its specificity of action on the serotonin system. It is useful in the treatment of major depressive disorder and may have special utility as a hypnotic in doses of 25 mg–50 mg at night. For this purpose, it can be an effective and nonaddicting alternative to the benzodiazepine hypnotics. It has fewer side effects than the TCAs for people who require pharmacological support of nonpharmacological treatments for the sleep disturbances of early recovery.

Carbamazepine has been shown to be useful in alcohol withdrawal states (82, 83). This drug, which is approved for use as an anticonvulsant, is also useful pharmacotherapy for people with affective disorders (84, 85). Because of its utility in withdrawal states, it is currently being investigated for use in maintaining abstinence in cocaine addicts (Brady, personal communication) and in my own work in alcohol dependence. Tegretol must be used cautiously by people on methadone maintenance as it may increase the metabolism of methadone and precipitate opioid withdrawal syndromes.

The benzodiazepines may be the most widely applied pharmacotherapy for major depressive disorder. Most of this prescribing occurs in the general medical setting and, in part, recognizes the high co-occurrence of anxiety symptoms with depressive syndromes. There is no clear evidence that the benzodiazepines are antidepressants (67). They are effective in treating the symptoms and complications of alcohol withdrawal but have no proven effectiveness in the long-term treatment of alcoholism or other drug dependence (86). There is as yet no resolution to the debate on whether benzodiazepines hold special abuse potential for people in early recovery; therefore, the weight of clinical evidence supports their use routinely only in withdrawal states (87).

6. *Electroconvulsive Treatment*

Electroconvulsive treatment (ECT) is an extremely effective and rapidly active treatment for major depressive disorder (88, 89). Its application in clinical populations has swung from wide usage when it was one of a few available somatic treatments, to a period of community-supported unpopularity, to its current utility in people with resistant depression, medical conditions, psychotic depression, and in the elderly (89–91). There is little literature evaluating the use of ECT in people recovering from chemical dependency. One study evaluating ECT in 58 people with secondary depression showed it to be effective in all of the five depressed alcoholics (92). My own experience with ECT has highlighted the challenges of diagnosing major depressive disorder in the setting of early recovery. What has been especially helpful in evaluating major depressive disorder and my application of ECT has been a longitudinal knowledge of the patient both personally and through the family. I have found it particularly effective in my patients with disabling depression who are not responding to conscientious efforts at abstinence and outpatient pharmacological treatment. It is extremely effective in terminating major depressive disorder. I have not found it useful in maintaining abstinence. Electroconvulsive treatment has some overlapping memory neurotoxicity with psychoactive chemicals of abuse, especially alcohol. Fortunately, the memory deficits that occur with ECT are transient. Nonetheless, after ECT, it is important to closely monitor and guard against the confusional states and attendant behavioral difficulty that can occur in the context of a memory disturbance.

C. Nonsomatic Treatments

There is little doubt that psychotherapy is helpful in treating major depressive disorder. It is in the identification of the active ingredients of these treatments where the challenge lies. Chapters 9, 10, and 11 describe the application of interpersonal psychotherapy, cognitive therapy, and problem solving therapy for patients with psychoactive substance abuse and dependence and depressive disorder. I will not elaborate on these treatments here. Not only are nonsomatic treatments helpful in major depressive disorder, but it appears that psychotherapy incrementally improves drug and alcohol treatment outcomes compared with standard treatments and improves psychiatric symptoms in people on methadone maintenance (93). There are two additional issues that I would like to address in this section—Alcoholics Anonymous and twelve-step treatment and family therapy.

1. Alcoholics Anonymous

Alcoholics Anonymous and twelve-step programs are the backbone of many recovering people's sobriety (94–96). Despite the historical acrimony between psychiatry and self-help programs, these treatments can powerfully aid depressed people as well as support abstinence. I am not aware of any specific evidence supporting the antidepressant efficacy of twelve-step programs, but they do contain many elements of effective psychotherapy. Alcoholics Anonymous provides a community of like-minded people, wherein people in early recovery can find camaraderie and social meaning. When a person in early recovery joins a group or obtains a sponsor, this establishes an immediate link with a community of supportive people. Bumper stickers such as ''A Friend of Bill W'' likewise reinforce the community identification that this treatment provides. This connection may "treat" the social isolation and loss of community meaning expressed by people in early recovery and identified as a theoretical model for depression (97). A lack of social support predicts the persistence of depressive symptoms in abstinent alcoholics (98). The AA meetings require only a willingness to stop drinking and do not require sobriety for attendance. This parallels the unconditional positive regard that is a powerful ingredient of most psychotherapies. Simple mottoes such as "One Day At a Time" and "Turn It Over," offer parallels to the "thought stopping" techniques that interrupt automatic dysfunctional thoughts in cognitive treatments. The serenity prayer and recitation of the Lord's Prayer provide a centering and focusing experience not uncommon to many hypnotic forms of treatment. The focus of AA on door prizes, medallions for successful periods of sobriety, and involvement in setting up and taking care of a meeting (making coffee), are fine examples of behaviorally oriented therapy. Step 4 of the Twelve Steps, when members undertake "a searching and fearless moral inventory," echoes many of the insight-oriented psychotherapies.

There are risks to AA. Historically, twelve-step programs have an antimedication, antiphysician, and antipsychiatry bias that can be powerful impediments to the dually diagnosed. Furthermore, the high co-occurrence of anxiety disorders among people with major depressive disorder can lead to situations in which untreated social phobias, obsessive compulsive disorder, panic attacks with or without agoraphobia, and post traumatic stress disorder can interfere with the effective use of the group modality. Nonetheless, that twelve-step programs contain many of the active ingredients of nonsomatic treatments for major depressive disorder may explain why AA has arrived at the conclusion that, in their extreme states, alcohol and drug abuse cause craziness, not the converse.

2. *Family Therapy*

The emergence and popularity of Al-Anon and similar groups illustrate the utility of involving family members and significant others in the treatment process. Despite the growth of these support groups and the wealth of evidence illustrating the effects of the addictions on family, there is little controlled empirical research on family treatments (99–101). Family function is affected by major depressive disorder, and family treatments are effective (102–104). The extant work suggests that family treatments have small beneficial effect in improving addiction treatment outcomes (105–108). Research on depressive populations with comorbid disorders (primarily psychoactive substance use disorders and medical problems) support the efficacy of family therapy in the treatment of depression in this group (109). The involvement of the family has been elaborated in networking therapy, which brings into abstinence-based treatment any identified significant individual in the recovering person's life (110). There may be some contraindications to this treatment as suggested in a recent study. It may be that people who have a low investment in social networks may not do well with treatments that rely on relationships (111). We need more systematic research in this area, evaluating the outcomes of family treatments on major depressive disorder in people in early recovery from addictions.

D. Unconventional Treatments

There is no focused data to evaluate the effectiveness of phototherapy or acupuncture in the treatment of major depressive disorder in early recovery. However, the finding that the addiction and recovery processes lead to disruption of people's normal life rhythms, as evidenced in sleep disturbance, suggests that phototherapy, which appears to be effective in reestablishing diurnal patterns in major depressive disorder, may be useful. The low cost and low toxicity of this modality further support this treatment as an area of further research (112, 113).

Acupuncture has a long history in far Eastern medicine. Its recent application in the Western world has been met with skepticism. Despite the difficulty in performing controlled experiments with acupuncture and designing sham acupuncture treatments, there is mixed but intriguing evidence that it may be effective in treating drug withdrawal states and supporting abstinence (114–116). Acupuncture is most typically used in acute and chronic pain syndromes. There is no report in the Western literature of its use in affective syndromes. However, it may have some utility in depressive states associated with pain syndromes in people in early recovery from alcohol and drug dependency (117, 118).

E. Human Immunodeficiency Virus Disease

Intravenous drug use and indiscriminate heterosexual behavior place psychoactive drug-using populations at increased risk for human immunodeficiency virus (HIV) disease. If current trends of increased HIV disease in drug-using populations continue, we will also see an increase in the psychiatric complications of HIV infection in recovering people. This infection is complicated by major depressive disorder in several ways. Primary central nervous system (CNS) infection has symptoms similar to major depressive disorder; CNS opportunistic infections can lead to major depressive disorder; and HIV typically has devastating life consequences that are associated with major depressive disorder (119, 120). People at risk for HIV infection also appear to have elevated risks for a lifetime history of mood disorders, exposing them to the possibility of a recurrence of affective syndromes (121). There are no unique recommendations for treatment of major depressive disorder in this population except for treatment of the HIV infection. However, the SSRIs, by virtue of their low side effect profile, may be preferable to TCAs in which the anticholinergic-related memory toxicity may aggravate HIV dementia syndromes (122). The TCAs do appear to be effective and do not compromise immune function (123).

F. Tobacco Dependence

Tobacco dependence is associated with depression. This has been demonstrated in both population surveys and in smoking cessation treatment outcome research (124, 125). In the United States, smokers report higher levels of depression than nonsmokers (126). There is preliminary evidence that the treatment of depression is useful in aiding attempts at smoking cessation. Doxepin, a TCA, has been shown to be effective in decreasing nicotine withdrawal syndromes, and preliminary evidence suggests that pretreatment with antidepressants may prevent the development of abstinence-related depressive syndromes in smokers with a history of major depressive disorder (127, 128).

Smokers with a history of major depressive disorder appear more likely to experience depressive symptoms and may be more likely to be unsuccessful in maintaining abstinence from tobacco use. There is no reason not to apply the broad range of previously described antidepressant treatments in this group. This is an area of active research. It is important to remember that smoking accelerates the metabolism of many drugs, including the TCAs (129).

G.   Other Addictive Behaviors

It is not widely accepted that other behaviors such as gambling and compulsive sexual activity represent addictions (130). However, this is an evolving area of clinical debate and scientific inquiry. People with psychoactive substance abuse and dependence have a high co-occurrence of pathological gambling (131). Also, the scant systematic literature that exists suggests that there are high levels of comorbid psychopathology, including depression, in people with pathological gambling and compulsive sexual activity (132–134). There is evidence that compulsive sexual activity and attendant depression symptoms respond to antidepressant pharmacotherapy (135, 136). Currently it appears that recommendations outlined earlier in this chapter for the treatment of major depressive disorder in early recovery from psychoactive substances also apply to the treatment of depression in these populations. The special attributes of treatment in these conditions are yet to be established.

H.   Conclusions

The treatment of major depressive disorder in early recovery is a challenging area for research and clinical practice. Despite an extensive literature, there are numerous gaps in our knowledge. Most of the research is done on men. We need to know more about women, especially in light of the fact that depression is more common in women than men by a ratio of two to one. There is also the tantalizing data that women alcoholics have more favorable outcomes if they are also depressed (43). There is a lack of research on long-term outcomes, that is, outcomes longer than a few months to one year. Until recently, little research concurrently monitored the activity of drug use and depressive symptoms. Earlier research was plagued by defects in methodology and few attempts to monitor drug levels and drug compliance. As we become more knowledgeable in this area, it will be useful to arrive at diagnostic criteria based on symptoms and phenomenology that recognize the overlap of the syndromes. We may at some point have the ability to use biological markers to aid in our diagnoses.

Ultimately, the application of treatments in major depressive disorder for people in early recovery is a cost/benefit equation. It is apparent that the cost of not diagnosing and treating major depressive disorder is extremely high in this population. Fortunately, the newer somatic treatments have low cost and high benefit, and sobriety based treatments and nonsomatic treatments appear to provide effective and overlapping activity for major depressive disorder and psychoactive substance abuse and dependence.

REFERENCES

1. J. A. Neff, Life stressors, drinking patterns and depressive symptomatology: Ethnicity and stress-buffer effects of alcohol, *Addictive Behaviors 18:*373–387 (1993).
2. S. L. Satel, T. R. Kosten, M. A. Schuckit, and M. W. Fischman, Should protracted withdrawal from drugs be included in DSM-IV?, *Am. J. Psychiatry 150:*695–704 (1993).
3. W. R. Yates, F. Petty, and K. Brown, Factors associated with depression among primary alcoholics, *Compr. Psych. 29:*28–33 (1988).
4. H. B. McNamee, N. K. Mello, and J. H. Mendelson, Experimental analysis of drinking patterns of alcoholics: Concurrent psychiatric observations, *Am. J. Psychiatry 124:*1063–1069 (1968).
5. J. S. Tamerin and J. H. Mendelson, The psychodynamics of chronic inebriation: Observations of alcoholics during the process of drinking in an experimental group setting, *Am. J. Psychiatry 125:*886–899 (1969).
6. F. H. Gawin and H. D. Kleber, Abstinence symptomatology and psychiatric diagnosis in cocaine abusers: Clinical observations, *Arch. Gen. Psychiatry 43:*107–113 (1986).
7. D. Behar, G. Winokur, and C. J. Berg, Depression in the abstinent alcoholic, *Am. J. Psychiatry, 141:*1105–1107 (1984).
8. D. Hatsukami and R. W. Dickens, Posttreatment depression in an alcohol and drug abuse population, *Am. J. Psychiatry 139:*1563–1566 (1982).

9. A. T. Butterworth, Depression associated with alcohol withdrawal, *Quart. J. Study Alc. 32:*343–348 (1971).
10. A. Blankfield, Psychiatric symptoms in alcohol dependence: Diagnostic and treatment implications, *J. Sub. Abuse Treatment 3:*275–278 (1986).
11. J. E. Zweben, and D. E. Smith, Considerations in using psychotropic medication with dual diagnosis patients in recovery. *J. Psychoactive Drugs 21:*221–228 (1989).
12. Alcoholics Anonymous, *The A.A. member—medications and other drugs. Alcoholics Anonymous World Services, Inc., New York City, 1984.*
13. H. W. Batson, L. S. Brown, A. R. Zaballero, A. Chu, and A. I. Alterman, Conflicting measurements of depression in a substance abuse population, *J. Substance Abuse 5:*93–100 (1993).
14. M. H. Keeler, C. I. Taylor, and W. C. Miller, Are all recently detoxified alcoholics depressed? *Am. J. Psychiatry, 136:*586–588 (1979).
15. R. D. Weiss, S. M. Mirin, M. L. Griffin, and J. L. Michael, Psychopathology in cocaine abusers *J. Nerv. and Mental Dis. 176:*719–725 (1988).
16. R. D. Weiss, M. L. Griffin and S. M. Mirin, Diagnosing major depression in cocaine abusers: The use of depression rating scales, *Psych. Res. 28:*335–343 (1989).
17. M. N. Hesselbrock, V. M. Hesselbrock, H. Tennen, R. E. Meyer, and K. L. Workman, Methodological considerations in the assessment of depression in alcoholics, *J. Consult. and Clin. Psych. 51:*399–405 (1983).
18. M. M. Kilbey, N. Breslau, and P. Andreski, Cocaine use and dependence in young adults: Associated psychiatric disorders and personality traits, *Drug and Alc. Dep. 29:*283–290 (1992).
19. D. A. Regier, M. E. Farmer, D. S. Rae, B. Z. Locke, S. J. Keith, L. L. Judd, and F. K. Goodwin, Comorbidity of mental disorders with alcohol and other drug abuse. *J.A.M.A. 264:*2511–2518 (1990).
20. M. M. Weissman, and J. K. Myers, Clinical depression in alcoholism, *Am. J. Psychiatry 137:*372–373 (1980).
21. E. J. Khantzian, The self-medication hypothesis of addictive disorders: Focus on heroin and cocaine dependence, *Am. J. Psychiatry 142:*1259–1264 (1985).
22. G. Winokur, Unipolar depression: Is it divisible into autonomous subtypes?, *Arch. Gen. Psychiatry 36:*47–52 (1979).
23. J. C. Ballenger and R. M. Post, Kindling as a model for alcohol withdrawal syndromes, *Brit. J. Psychiatry 133:*1–14 (1978).

24. R. M. Post, Transduction of psychosocial stress into the neurobiology of recurrent affective disorder, *Am. J. Psychiatry 149:*999–1010 (1992).

25. C. R. Cloninger, Neurogenetic adaptive mechanisms in alcoholism, *Science 236:*410–416 (1987).

26. K. R. Merikangas, J. F. Leckman, B. A. Prusoff, D. L. Pauls, and M. M. Weissman, Familial transmission of depression and alcoholism, *Arch. Gen. Psychiatry 42:*367–372 (1985).

27. M. A. Schuckit, Genetic and clinical implications of alcoholism and affective disorder, *Am. J. Psychiatry 143:*140–147 (1986).

28. K. S. Kendler, A. C. Heath, M. C. Neale, R. C. Kessler, and L. J. Eaves, Alcoholism and major depression in women: A twin study of the causes of comorbidity, *Arch. Gen. Psychiatry 50:*690–698 (1993).

29. R. Z. Litten and J. P. Allen, Pharmacotherapies for alcoholism: Promising agents and clinical issues, *Alcoholism: Clin. Exp. Res. 15:*620–633 (1991).

30. J. E. Turnbull and E. S. L. Gomberg, The structure of depression in alcoholic women, *J. Stud. Alc. 51:*148–155 (1990).

31. M. Schuckit, Alcoholic patients with secondary depression, *Am. J. Psychiatry 140:*711–714 (1983).

32. K. Hasegawa, H. Mukasa, Y. Nakazawa, H. Kodama, and K. Kakamura, Primary and secondary depression in alcoholism—clinical features and family history, *Drug and Alc. Dep. 27:*275–281 (1991).

33. M. A. Schuckit and M. G. Monteiro, Alcoholism, anxiety and depression, *Brit. J. Addiction 83:*1373–1380 (1988).

34. F. Petty, The depressed alcoholic: Clinical features and medical management, *Gen. Hosp. Psychiatry 14:*258–264 (1992).

35. K. O'Sullivan, C. Rynne, J. Miller, V. Fitzpatrick, M. Hux, J. Cooney, and A. Clare, A followup study on alcoholics with and without co-existing affective disorder, *Brit. J. Psych. 152:*813–819 (1988).

36. K. O'Sullivan, P. Whillans, M. Daly, B. Carroll, A. Clare, and J. Cooney, A comparison of alcoholics with and without coexisting affective disorder, *Brit. J. Psychiatry 143:*133–138 (1983).

37. E. Nunes, ''Depression in substance abusers: Evaluation and treatment,'' Presented at the Fourth Annual Symposium, the American Academy of Psychiatrists in Alcoholism and Addictions, Palm Beach, Florida, December 1993.

38. M. B. Keller, P. W. Lavori, G. Klerman, N. C. Andreasen, J. Endicott, W. Coryell, J. Fawcett, and R. M. A. Hirschfeld, Low levels and lack of predictors of somatotherapy and psychotherapy received by depressed patients, *Arch. Gen. Psychiatry 43:*458–466 (1986).

39. M. Pottenger, J. McKernon, L. E. Patrie, M. M. Weissman, H. L. Ruben, and P. Newberry, The frequency and persistence of depressive symptoms in the alcohol abuser, *J. Nerv. Ment. Dis. 166:*562–570 (1978).

40. G. E. Murphy, R. D. Wetzel, E. Robins, and L. McEvoy, Multiple risk factors predict suicide in alcoholism, *Arch. Gen. Psychiatry 49:*459–463 (1992).

41. J. P. MacMurray, D. G. Nessman, M. G. Haviland, and D. L. Anderson, Depressive symptoms and persistence in treatment for alcohol dependence, *J. Stud. Alcohol. 48:*277–280 (1987).

42. A. T. McLellan, L. Luborsky, G. E. Woody, C. P. O'Brien, and K. A. Druley, Predicting response to alcohol and drug abuse treatments, *Alcohol and Drug Abuse 40:*620–625 (1982).

43. B. J. Rounsaville, Z. S. Dolinsky, T. F. Babor, and R. E. Meyer, Psychopathology as a predictor of treatment outcome in alcoholics, *Arch. Gen. Psychiatry 44:*505–513 (1987).

44. K. M. Carroll, M. E. D. Power, K. Bryant, and B. J. Rounsaville, One-year follow-up status of treatment-seeking cocaine abusers: Psychopathology and dependence severity as predictors of outcome, *J. Nerv. Ment. Dis. 181:*71–79 (1993).

45. R. M. A. Hirschfeld, T. Kosier, M. B. Keller, P. W. Lavori, and S. Endicott, The influence of alcoholism on the course of depression, *J. Affect. Disord. 16:*151–158 (1989).

46. T. I. Mueller, P. W. Lavori, M. B. Keller, A. Swartz, M. Warshaw, D. Hasin, W. Coryell, J. Endicott, J. Rice, and H. Akiskal, The prognostic effect of the variable course of alcoholism on the 10-year course of depression, *Am. J. Psychiatry* In press, (1994).

47. K. O'Sullivan, Depression and its treatment in alcoholics: A review, *Can. J. Psychiatry, 29:*379–384 (1984).

48. G. I. Keitner and I. W. Miller, Combined psychopharmacological and psychosocial treatment for depression, *R. I. Medicine 76:*415–424 (1993).

49. American Psychiatric Association, Practice guideline for major depressive disorder in adults, *Am. J. Psychiatry 150 (suppl):*1–23 (1993).

50. S. A. Cohen-Cole, F. W. Brown, and J. S. McDaniel, Assessment of depression and grief reactions in the medically ill, *In: Psychiatric care of the medical patient* (A. Stoudemire, and B. S. Fogel, eds.), Oxford University Press, New York, 1993 pp. 53–70.

51. E. C. Strain, M. I. Stitzer, and G. E. Bigelow, Early treatment time course of depressive symptoms in opiate addicts, *J. Nerv. Ment. Dis. 178:*215–221 (1991).

52. S. A. Brown and M. A. Schuckit, Changes in depression among abstinent alcoholics, *J. Stud. Alc 49:*412–417 (1988).

53. H. M. Pettinati, A. A. Sugerman, N. DiDonato, and H. S. Maurer, The natural history of alcoholism over four years after treatment, *J. Stud. Alcohol. 42:*201–215 (1982).

54. M. M. Nakamura, J. E. Overall, L. E. Hollister, and E. Radcliffe, Factors affecting outcome of depressive symptoms in alcoholics, *Alcoholism: Clin. Exp. Res. 7:*188–193 (1983).

55. D. F. Klein, R. Gittelman, F. Quitkin, and A. Rifkin, *Diagnosis and drug treatment of psychiatric disorders: Adults and children,* 2nd ed. Williams and Wilkins, Baltimore, MD, 1980.

56. J. A. Shaw, P. Donley, D. W. Morgan, and J. A. Robinson, Treatment of depression in alcoholics, *Am. J. Psychiatry 132:*641–644 (1975).

57. J. E. Overall, D. Brown, J. D. Williams, and L. T. Neill, Drug treatment and anxiety and depression in detoxified alcoholic patients, *Arch. Gen. Psychiatry 29:*218–221 (1973).

58. A. T. Butterworth and R. D. Watts, Treatment of hospitalized alcoholics with doxepin and diazepam: A controlled study, *Quart. J. Stud. Alc. 32:*78–81 (1971).

59. I. C. Wilson, L. B. Alltop, and L. Riley, Tofranil in the treatment of post alcoholic depressions, *Psychosomatics 11:*488–494 (1970).

60. R. D. Weiss and S. M. Mirin, Tricyclic antidepressants in the treatment of alcoholism and drug abuse, *J. Clin. Psychiatry 50:*4–11 (1989).

61. D. A. Ciraulo and J. H. Jaffe, Tricyclic antidepressants in the treatment of depression associated with alcoholism, *J. Clin. Psychopharmacol. 1:*146–150 (1981).

62. I. O. Arndt, L. Dorozynsky, G. E. Woody, A. T. McLellan, and C. P. O'Brien, Desipramine treatment of cocaine dependence in methadone-maintained patients, *Arch. Gen. Psychiatry 39:*888–893 (1992).

63. B. J. Mason and J. H. Kocsis, Desipramine treatment of alcoholism, *Psychopharmacology Bulletin 27:*155–161 (1991).

64. E. V. Nunes, P. J. McGrath, F. M. Quitkin, J. P. Stewart, W. Harrison, E. Tricamo, and K. Ocepek-Welikson, Imipramine treatment of alcoholism with comorbid depression, *Am. J. Psychiatry 150:*963–965 (1993).

65. D. A. Ciraulo, L. M. Alderson, D. J. Chapron, J. H. Jaffe, B. Subbarao, and P. A. Kramer, Imipramine disposition in alcoholics, *J. Clin. Psychopharmacol. 2:*2–7 (1982).

66. R. S. Schottenfield, S. S. O'Malley, L. Smith, B. J. Rounsaville, and J. H. Jaffe, Clinical note: Limitation and potential hazards of MAOI's for the treatment of depressive symptoms in abstinent alcoholics, *Am. J. Drug Alcohol Abuse 15:*339–344 (1989).

67. M. R. Liebowitz, Depression with anxiety and atypical depression, *J. Clin. Psychiatry 54:*2 (suppl) 10–14 (1993).
68. M. R. Liebowitz, and D. F. Klein, Hysteroid dysphoria, *Psychiatric Clin. N. America 2:*555–575 (1979).
69. F. M. Quitkin, A. Rifkin, and D. F. Klein, Monoamine oxidase inhibitors: A review of antidepressant effectiveness, *Arch. Gen. Psychiatry 36:*749–760 (1979).
70. J. Fawcett, D. C. Clark, R. D. Gibbons, C. A. Aagesen, V. D. Pisani, J. M. Tilkin, D. Sellers, and D. Stutzman, Evaluation of lithium therapy for alcoholism, *J. Clin. Psychiatry 45:*494–499 (1984).
71. N. S. Kline, J. C. Wren, T. B. Cooper, E. Varga, and O. Canal, Evaluation of lithium therapy in chronic and periodic alcoholism, *Am. J. Med. Sci. 268:*15–22 (1974).
72. J. Merry, C. M. Reynolds, J. Bailey, and A. Coppen, Prophylactic treatment of alcoholism by lithium corbonate: A controlled study, *Lancet 2:*481–482 (1976).
73. L. L. Judd and L. Y. Huey, Lithium antagonizes lithium intoxication in alcoholics, *Am. J. Psychiatry 141:*1517–1521 (1984).
74. W. Dorus, D. G. Ostrow, R. Anton, P. Cushman, J. F. Collins, M. Schaefer, H. L. Charles, P. Desai, M. Hayashida, U. Malkerneker, M. Willenbring, R. Fiscella, and M. Sather, Lithium treatment of depressed and nondepressed alcoholics, *J.A.M.A. 262:*1646–1652 (1989).
75. C. DéMontigny, F. Grunberg, A. Mayer, and J. P. Deschenes, Lithium induces rapid relief of depression in tricyclic antidepressant drug nonresponders, *Brit. J. Psychiatry 138:*252–256 (1981).
76. T. F. Meert, Effects of various serotonergic agents on alcohol intake and alcohol preference in wistar rats selected at two different levels of alcohol preference, *Alcohol and Alcoholism 28:*157–170 (1993).
77. E. D. Levin, S. J. Briggs, N. C. Christopher, and J. E. Rose, Sertraline attenuates hyperphagia in rats following nicotine withdrawal, *Pharmacology, Biochemistry and Behavior 44:*51–61 (1993).
78. D. H. Overstreet, A. H. Rezvani, and D. S. Janowsky, Genetic animal models of depression and ethanol preference provide support for cholinergic and serotonergic involvement in depression and alcoholism, *Biol. Psychiatry 31:*919–936 (1992).
79. C. A. Naranjo, K. E. Kadlec, P. Sanhueza, D. Woodley-Remus, and E. M. Sellers, Fluoxetine differentially alters alcohol intake and other consummatory behaviors in problem drinkers, *Clin. Pharmacol. Ther. 47:*490–498 (1990).
80. B. E. Leonard. The comparative pharmacology of new antidepressants, *J. Clin. Psychiatry 54:*(suppl) 3–15 (1993).

81. P. D. Kramer, *Listening to Prozac*, Viking, New York, (1993).
82. R. Malcolm, J. C. Ballenger, E. T. Sturgis, and R. Anton, Double-blind controlled trial comparing carbamazepine to oxazepam treatment of alcohol withdrawal, *Am. J. Psychiatry 5:*617–621 (1989).
83. D. Butler and F. S. Messiha, Alcohol withdrawal and carbamazepine, *Alcohol 3:*113–129 (1986).
84. R. M. Post, D. R. Rubinow, and T. W. Uhde, Biochemical mechanisms of action of carbamazepine in affective illness and epilepsy, *Psychopharmacology Bulletin 20:*585–589 (1984).
85. R. M. Post, S. R. B. Weiss, and D. Chuang, Mechanisms of action of anticonvulsants in affective disorders: Comparisons with lithium, *J. Clin. Psychopharmacol. 12:*23S–35S (1992).
86. D. Nutt, B. Adinoff, and M. Linnoila, Benzodiazepines in the treatment of alcoholism. *In: Recent Developments in Alcoholism,* Volume 7, Treatment Research, (M. Galanter, ed.) Plenum Press, New York, 1989.
87. D. A. Ciraulo, B. F. Sands, and R. I. Shader, Critical review of liability for benzodiazepine abuse among alcoholics, *Am. J. Psychiatry 145:* 1501–1506 (1988).
88. M. W. Enns and J. P. Reiss, Electroconvulsive therapy, *Can. J. Psychiatry 37:*671–678 (1992).
89. K. Persad, Electroconvulsive therapy in depression, *Can. J. Psychiatry 35:*175–182 (1990).
90. B. S. Fogel, Electroconvulsive therapy in the elderly: A clinical research agenda, *Intl. J. Geriatric Psych. 3:*181–190 (1988).
91. B. L. Selvin, Electroconvulsive therapy—1987, *Anesthesiology 67:*367–385 (1987).
92. C. F. Zorumski, J. L. Rutherford, W. J. Burke, and T. Reich, ECT in primary and secondary depression, *J. Clin. Psychiatry 47:*298–300 (1986).
93. A. T. McLellan, I. O. Arndt, D. S. Metzger, G. E. Woody, and C. P. O'Brien, The effects of psychosocial services in substance abuse treatment, *J.A.M.A. 15:*1953–1959 (1993).
94. Alcoholics Anonymous, *Twelve steps and twelve traditions,* Alcoholics Anonymous World Services, Inc., New York City, 1953.
95. M. Galanter, Cults and zealous self-help movements: A psychiatric perspective, *Am. J. Psychiatry 147:*543–551 (1990).
96. J. N. Chappel, Effective use of alcoholics anonymous and narcotics anonymous in treating patients, *Psychiatric Annals 22:*409–418 (1992).
97. P. Gilbert, *Depression: The evolution of powerlessness,* The Guilford Press, New York, 1992.
98. J. E. Overall, E. L. Reilly, J. T. Kelley, and L. E. Hollister, Persistence

of. depression in detoxified alcoholics, *Alcoholism: Clin. Exp. Res.* *9*:331–333 (1985).

99.   B. S. McCrady, Outcomes of family-involved alcoholism treatment, *In: Recent Developments in Alcoholism,* Volume 7, treatment research, (M. Galanter, ed.), Plenum Press, New York, (1989).

100. M. R. Liepman, L. Y. Silvia, and T. D. Nirenberg, The use of family behavior loop mapping for substance abuse, *Family Relations 38*:282–287 (1989).

101. J. K. Jackson, The adjustment of the family to the crisis of alcoholism, *Quarterly. J. Stud. Alc. 4*:562–586 (1954).

102. G. I. Keitner, I. W. Miller, N. B. Epstein, D. S. Bishop, and A. E. Fruzzetti, Family functioning and the course of major depression, *Compr. Psych. 28*:54–64 (1987).

103. J. H. Spencer, I. D. Glick, G. L. Haas, J. F. Clarkin, A. B. Lewis, J. Peyser, N. DeMane, M. Good-Ellis, E. Harris, and V. Lestelle, A randomized clinical trial of inpatient family intervention, III: Effects at 6-month and 18-month follow-ups, *Am. J. Psychiatry 9*:1115–1121 (1988).

104. G. I. Keitner and I. W. Miller, Family functioning and major depression: An overview, *Am. J. Psychiatry 147:* 1128–1137 (1990).

105. T. J. O'Farrell, Marital and family therapy in alcoholism treatment, *J. Substance Abuse Treatment 6*:23–29 (1989).

106. B. E. Mapes, R. A. Johnson, and K. R. Sandler, The alcoholic family: Diagnosis and treatment, *Alcoholism Treatment Quarterly 4*:67–83 (1984).

107. M. R. Liepman, T. D. Nirenberg, and W. T. White, Family-oriented treatment of alcoholism, *R. I. Medical Journal 68*:123–126 (1985).

108. M. R. Liepman, T. D. Nirenberg, R. H. Doolittle, A. M. Begin, T. E. Broffman, and M. E. Babich, Family functioning of male alcoholics and their female partners during periods of drinking and abstinence, *Family Process 2*:239–249 (1989).

109. B. M. Booth, D. W. Russell, W. R. Yates, P. R. Laughlin, K. Brown, and D. Reed, Social support and depression in men during alcoholism treatment, *J. Substance Abuse 4*:57–67 (1992).

110. M. Galanter, Network therapy for addiction: A model for office practice, *Am. J. Psychiatry 150*:28–36 (1993).

111. R. Longabaugh, M. Beattie, N. Noel, R. Stout, and P. Malloy, The effect of social investment on treatment outcome, *J. Stud. Alc.* 465–478 (1993).

112. R. W. Lam, D. F. Kripke, and J. C. Gillin, Phototherapy for depressive disorders: A review, *Can. J. Psychiatry 34*:140–147 (1989).

113. C. A. Czeisler, R. E. Kronauer, J. J. Mooney, J. L. Anderson, and J. S. Allan, Biologic rhythm disorders, depression, and phototherapy: A new hypothesis, *Psychiatric Clin. North Am. 10:*687–709 (1987).

114. A. G. Brumbaugh, Acupuncture: New perspectives in chemical dependency treatment, *J. Substance Abuse Treatment 10:*35–43 (1993).

115. T. M. Worner, B. Zeller, H. Schwarz, F. Zwas, and D. Lyon, Acupuncture fails to improve treatment outcome in alcoholics, *Drug and Alcohol Dependence 30:*169–173 (1992).

116. A. Margolin, S. K. Avants, P. Chang, and T. R. Kosten, Acupuncture for the treatment of cocaine dependence in methadone-maintained patients, *Am. J. Addictions 2:*194–201 (1993).

117. K. Kuch, B. Cox, R. J. Evans, P. C. Watson, and C. Bubela, To what extent do anxiety and depression interact with chronic pain? *Can. J. Psychiatry 38:*36–38 (1993).

118. S. Tyrer, Psychiatric assessment of chronic pain, *Brit. J. Psychiatry 160:*733–741 (1992).

119. S. Tross and D. A. Hirsch, Psychological distress and neuropsychological complications of HIV infection and AIDS, *American Psychologist 43:*929–934 (1988).

120. S. W. Perry, Organic mental disorders caused by HIV: Update on early diagnosis and treatment, *Am. J. Psychiatry 147:*679–710 (1990).

121. S. Perry, L. B. Jacobsberg, B. Fishman, A. Frances, J. Bobo, and B. K. Jacobsberg, Psychiatric diagnosis before serological testing for the human immunodeficiency virus, *Am. J. Psychiatry 147:*89–93 (1990).

122. D. O. Perkins and D. L. Evans, Fluoxetine treatment of depression in patients with HIV infection (Letter), *Am. J. Psychiatry 148:*807–808 (1991).

123. J. G. Rabkin and W. M. Harrison, Effect of imipramine on depression and immune status in a sample of men with HIV infection, *Am. J. Psychiatry 147:*495–497 (1990).

124. R. A. Brown, M. G. Goldstein, R. Niaura, K. M. Emmons, and D. B. Abrams, Nicotine dependence: Assessment and management, (A. Stoudemire, and B. S. Fogel, eds.), *Psychiatric Care of the Medical Patient,* Oxford Press, New York (1993).

125. L. S. Covey, A. H. Glassman, and F. Stetner, Depression and depressive symptoms in smoking cessation, *Compr. Psychiatry 31:*350–354 (1990).

126. A. H. Glassman, Cigarette smoking: Implications for psychiatric illness, *Am. J. Psychiatry 150:* 546–553 (1993).

127. N. B. Edwards, J. K. Murphy, A. D. Downs, B. J. Ackerman, and T. L. Roenthal, Antidepressants as an adjunct to smoking cessation: A double-blind study, *Am. J. Psychiatry 146:*373–376 (1989).

128. A. H. Glassman, L. S. Covey, and F. Stener, Smoking cessation, depression and antidepressants, Presented at the annual meeting of the American Psychiatric Association, San Francisco, CA, May, 1989.

129. N. L. Benowitz, Pharmacologic aspects of cigarette smoking and nicotine addiction. *N. Engl. J. Med. 319:*1318–1330 (1988).

130. S. L. Satel, The diagnostic limits of "addiction," (Letter), *J. Clin. Psychiatry 54:*237 (1993).

131. H. R. Lesieur and S. B. Blume, Evaluation of patients treated for pathological gambling in a combined alcohol, substance abuse and pathological gambling treatment unit using the Addiction Severity Index, *Brit. J. Addiction 86:*1017–1028 (1991).

132. R. A. McCormick, Disinhibition and negative affectivity in substance abusers with and without a gambling problem, *Addictive Behaviors 18:*331–336 (1993).

133. S. Legg England and K. G. Götestam, The nature and treatment of excessive gambling. *Acta Psychiatr. Scand. 84:*113–120 (1991).

134. M. P. Kafka, Successful antidepressant treatment of nonparaphilic sexual addictions and paraphilias in men, *J. Clin. Psychiatry 52:*60–65 (1991).

135. M. P. Kafka and R. Prentky, Fluoxetine treatment of nonparaphilic sexual addictions and paraphilias in men, *J. Clin. Psychiatry 53:*351–358 (1992).

136. D. J. Stein, E. Hollander, D. T. Anthony, F. R. Schneier, B. A. Fallon, M. R. Liebowitz, and D. F. Klein, Serotonergic medications for sexual obsessions, sexual addictions, and paraphilias, *J. Clin. Psychiatry 53:*267–271 (1992).

5

Treatment of Dysthymia

Raymond L. Ownby and Barbara J. Mason
University of Miami School of Medicine, Miami, Florida

I. INTRODUCTION

Many recovering addicts present a diagnostic and treatment dilemma to the clinician supervising their treatment: They may present multiple symptoms of depression but not meet full criteria for a major depressive episode. It is difficult at times to know whether the condition is of sufficient severity to merit treatment. This dilemma is further complicated by the question of whether the depressive symptoms are long-standing (and the addiction was an unfortunate attempt at self-treatment) or recent (and thus may arise from the addiction itself). Clinicians have been advised to treat or not to treat these symptoms in recovering addicts, depending on the resolution of this dilemma.

Those treating recovering addicts must also address a persistent problem in the area of mood disorders: What is the nature of minor chronic depression, and when is treatment (either pharmacological or psychotherapeutic) likely to be successful? Various authors have argued for the existence of multiple subtypes of minor depression; clinical lore and some empirical research exist to validate these subtypes, whose importance rests in the putative susceptibility of each to treatment. In this chapter, we will address this diagnostic problem as a *cross-sectional* issue. To clarify the diagnostic issue, it is important to decide whether a particular constellation of symptoms exists in the patient at a given point in time.

In addressing this question, those treating recovering addicts also address a persistent controversy in theory about the etiology of mood disorders among addicts. Did the mood disorder exist before the addiction, and did the addiction represent an attempt by the addict to self-treat symptoms with mood altering substances? This is a question that requires *longitudinal* information about the time course of mood symptoms, especially in relation to the addiction. Some empirical data exist on this issue, at least in groups of recovering addicts. These data suggest that the overlap between groups of people with mood disorders and with addictions may be smaller than often thought.

A final concern for the clinician, in contrast to the researcher on mood disorders and addictions, is whether the mood symptoms presented by the recovering addict merit treatment. Traditional approaches taken by some twelve-step programs proscribe the use of psychoactive medication, but more recent thought has recognized the potential importance of treatment of mood disorders in recovering addicts. Once the clinician has decided that treatment is indicated, a variety of interventions are available, and it is possible that some combination of pharmacological and psychotherapeutic strategies may be optimal for individual patients.

In this chapter, we review how to approach patients with minor depressive symptoms. How does the clinician decide whether a treatable mood disorder is present? We will also review evidence on the relation of mood disorders and addictions and hope to clarify this relation with specific attention to the presence of mood symptoms in recovering addicts. Finally, we will address treatment choice for mood symptoms, and the possibility that combined treatments may be useful in this clinical situation.

II. DYSTHYMIA

Researchers have long recognized that many patients may present with multiple symptoms of depression that, when taken together, do not constitute an episode of major depression. One of the most persistent controversies in this area has been whether chronic mild depression represents a personality disorder or a mood disorder. Traditional thinking has emphasized the personality disorder theory, and consistent with traditional thought, the poor prognosis of such patients has also been emphasized. More recently, however, researchers have shown a connection between such patients and relatives with other, more explicitly syndromic, mood disorders. This finding suggests that persons with chronic mild depressive symptoms may present with a true mood disorder that could be expected to be amenable to the same treatments as are other mood disorders.

As noted by Akiskal (1), "The need for the 'dysthymia' construct arose because of the existence of a large spectrum of patients with fluctuating, intermittent, or chronic depression . . ." The Diagnostic and Statistical Manual-4th Edition (DSM-IV) defines dysthymic disorder as comprising "a chronically depressed mood that occurs for most of the day more days than not for at least 2 years." (2) "During periods of depressed mood, at least two of the following additional symptoms are present: poor appetite or overeating, insomnia or hypersomnia, low energy or fatigue, low self-esteem, poor concentration or difficulty making decisions, and feeling of hopelessness." (2) A hallmark of the disorder is its chronicity: "Because these symptoms become so much a part of the individual's day-to-day experience (e.g., 'I've always been this way,' 'That's just how I am'), they are often not reported (3).

Some authors believe that the symptoms listed overemphasize the similarity between major depression and dysthymia, by including vegetative symptoms of depression, such as disturbances in sleep and appetite. They have argued for an alternative set of diagnostic criteria for dysthymia that stresses subjective aspects of the disorder, such as low self-confidence, hopelessness, and feelings of irritability or being easily angered. This alternate conceptualization of dysthymia is codified in a set of research criteria for dysthymia in DSM-IV (4).

In DSM-IV as well, describing the patient's symptoms further is possible according to their similarity to "atypical depression." Atypical depression refers to a constellation of symptoms sometimes seen in depressed patients, including hypersomnia, excessive appetite, sensitivity to interpersonal rejection, and feelings of leaden paralysis in the legs. Research suggests that patients with this form of major depression may respond better to monamine oxidase inhibitors (MAOIs) or serotonin-specific reuptake inhibitors (SSRIs), as opposed to tricyclic antidepressants (TCAs). It is possible that dysthymic patients with this pattern of symptoms may show a similar pattern of response.

The differential diagnosis of dysthymia is broad and includes a wide range of depressive, psychotic, and substance-induced disorders, as well as disorders due to medical conditions and their treatments. Here we will focus only on the DSM-IV disorders most closely related to dysthymia. These include substance-induced mood disorders, cyclothymic disorder, and depressive disorder not otherwise specified. Subsumed in this last disorder are several subtypes of depression thought by some researchers to exist, but that have not been well researched. These are: 1) brief recurrent depression, in which patients experience full-blown episodes of depression that do not last a sufficient length of time to be considered a major depressive disorder; 2) minor depression, in which patients experience depressive symptoms that do not meet criteria for major depression, but in which the symptoms are less chronic than in dysthymia. Dysthymia may also be distinguished from depressive personality disorder, considered by some to be a chronic pattern of personality function characterized by a gloomy mood and beliefs of inadequacy (5). It should be noted that most of these subtypes of depressive disorders are not well researched, and ultimately, treatment decisions may depend more on the patient's clinical picture at the time of presentation than on more precise diagnosis.

Perhaps the single most important diagnostic issue confronting the clinician who works with addicts in various phases of recovery is the relation of the patient's mood symptoms to substance abuse. This consideration may be especially important in the early phases of recovery, when depressive symptoms are common and may result from biochemical and psychological factors.

For nonmedical clinicians, the issue may be the extent to which depressive symptoms should be the focus of psychotherapeutic interventions. Later in treatment, the clinician may also be confronted with mood symptoms persisting after a period of treatment, causing concern about whether pharmacological treatment is indicated. The medical clinician faces these concerns, as well as whether to initiate pharmacological interventions at the outset of treatment. Conventional wisdom suggests that antidepressant therapy is not indicated for depressive symptoms in the immediate recovery period, because these often resolve spontaneously. The severity of such early recovery depression, however, may lead the clinician to initiate pharmacological and psychotherapeutic treatment immediately, rather than risk delay in treating a potentially disabling depression.

A. Assessment

Assessment of dysthymia in the recovering addict should focus on the pattern of symptoms present and their severity and chronicity. Assessing the symptoms listed in the alternate criteria for dysthymia may also be useful, as discussed above. Finally, a determination of the presence of atypical depressive symptoms may also help guide therapeutic efforts.

Assessment of severity of symptoms should focus on the impact of dysthymic symptoms on patients' present and past functioning. This impact should be assessed not only in relation to social and vocational functioning, but also in personal functioning. Some patients with clinically significant dysthymia may function well daily but experience mood symptoms that significantly interfere with their life satisfaction. Assessment should therefore investigate not only the impact of dysthymic symptoms on vocational and social functioning, but should also focus more broadly on the impact of the symptoms on the patient's ability to enjoy life. For example, the patient may have been successful at a job for many years but might describe himself or herself as completely miserable during the time. Such a situation might also be related to the development of a substance abuse problem, and a failure to address it might be related to relapse. The patient's quality of life and more general behavioral functioning should be an object of clinical assessment and treatment.

B. Treatment

Treatment of dysthymia involves a judicious selection of several therapeutic modalities. These include pharmacotherapy, psychotherapy, or some combination of both. Although the development of knowledge on the best ways to treat dysthymia is in its early stages, enough information exists to suggest that some medications may be more effective than others in the treatment of dysthymia. Similarly, information exists that suggests that some forms of psychotherapy may be more effective than others. The clinician's task is to assess the patient's symptoms and determine whether treatment is indicated. If treatment is indicated, then the clinician should decide what combination of psychotherapeutic and pharmacotherapeutic strategies is indicated.

Although this determination will inevitably be a matter of clinical judgment, a few broad guidelines can be advanced. Perhaps the single most important factor in treatment choice for dysthymia will be severity of symptoms. It may be advisable to choose, at least as part of an initial treatment strategy, pharmacotherapy when the patient's symptoms are chronic and severe. This may be especially true when the symptoms interfere with social or occupational functioning or when they appear to affect the patient's risk for relapse into addiction. By contrast, psychotherapy alone may be a single initial treatment when symptoms are mild and have a clear cognitive component likely to be addressable in verbal psychotherapy (especially such therapies as cognitive-behavioral therapy or interpersonal psychotherapy). The clinician will probably encounter some patients who would prefer not to take medications for control of their symptoms; this group may also be initially treated with psychotherapy alone. Dysthymic symptoms with a more strongly vegetative component (e.g., sleep or appetite disturbance, lack of energy, sexual dysfunction) may respond to pharmacotherapy. Persistent dysthymic symptoms that do not respond to a reasonable trial of psychotherapy should also be addressed with a trial of antidepressant medication.

What follows is a brief review of illustrative studies on treatment strategies for dysthymia. Although it is possible that pharmacotherapy alone may be the single treatment for a recovering addict with dysthymia, it is hard to imagine circumstances in which the addict would not also present with significant personal and social issues. These probably should be addressed in psychotherapy in some manner. It is also likely that a patient with dysthymia, by definition a chronic condition, may also present with psychosocial issues that should be addressed in psychotherapy.

1. Pharmacotherapy

Several medications have been used to treat dysthymia, including tricyclic agents, SSRIs, MAOIs, and reversible inhibitors of monoamine oxidase (RIMAs). Although one combined serotonergic and noradrenergic reuptake inhibitor is currently available in the United States (venlafaxine), we know of no studies that have investigated treatment of dysthymia with it. Although clinical lore had long caused pessimistic attitudes toward the treatment of dysthymia, most studies have shown that an important proportion of dysthymic patients may respond to pharmacotherapy.

a. Tricyclic Antidepressants. Several studies have investigated the use of TCAs for dysthymic patients. Kocsis et al. (6) found in a double-blind, placebo-controlled trial of imipramine in chronic depression that 59% of study completers showed significant improvement in depressive symptoms that they had experienced for many years. By contrast, only 13% of study completers on a placebo showed substantial response. In addition, these authors noted that most of these patients also fulfilled DSM-III criteria for major depression and had been untreated or undertreated for lengthy periods before their entry in the study. This study is of interest for several reasons, the most salient of which is its clear demonstration of the effectiveness of antidepressant medication in the treatment of dysthymia. It is also of interest for its demonstration of a low placebo response rate in this group of patients, suggesting the importance of pharmacotherapy for the disorder. Kocsis et al. (7) also reported significant improvement in these patients' social and vocational performance after treatment. In a follow-up study, Kocsis et al. (8) showed that predicting response of dysthymic patients to treatment was not possible. In this study, treatment outcome was not related to demographic variables, severity or course of depression, depressive subtype, pattern of symptoms, or results of the dexamethasone suppression test. Similar findings supporting the use of imipramine for treatment of dysthymia are reported by Bakish et al. (9) in a comparison of imipramine with ritanserin (see discussion of ritanserin below).

Marin et al. (10) report an 8-week open trial of desipramine, comparing its effectiveness in patients meeting diagnostic criteria for both dysthymia and major depression (''double depression'') vs. those with dysthymia alone. Complete or partial remission of symptoms was achieved by 70% of the dysthymic patients, whereas 52% of the patients with double depression had achieved complete or partial remission by the end of the study. Although this difference appears substantial, it was not statistically significant. It should also be noted that this was a short trial of medication for major depression.

Other studies have suggested that various TCAs may be useful in dysthymia, but these are not reviewed here because of limitations in diagnosis or research methodology. For example, Kornhaber and Horwitz (11) showed that both clomipramine and doxepin may be effective in ''neurotic depression.'' This study, however, used a DSM-II diagnostic category with an uncertain relation to the current diagnosis of dysthymia. Similarly, Paykel et al. (12) showed that amitriptyline (and phenelzine) may be effective in subtypes of depression potentially related to dysthymia, but assessing diagnostic overlap in this study is difficult.

The response of major depression in alcoholic patients to TCAs has been investigated in several studies (13;14). Mason and Kocsis showed that depression among alcoholics responded to desipramine, whereas Nunes et al. showed that depression may respond to imipramine. Mason and Kocsis also showed that relapse was more likely in depressed alcoholics who were randomly assigned to a placebo control group. Although these studies are not directly related to the treatment of dysthymia, they show that a similar disorder, major depression, may respond to TCA treatment in a population of alcohol abusers. Results of the Mason and Kocsis study also show the possibly greater risk of relapse among depressed patients who are trying to achieve abstinence, but whose depression is not adequately treated.

b. Monoamine Oxidase Inhibitors. The only MAOI systematically studied in dysthymia is phenelzine. Perhaps stimulated by studies showing the effectiveness of MAOIs in atypical depression (15), Stewart et al. (16) showed a significant response of chronic depression to phenelzine. Vallejo et al. (17) showed that both imipramine and phenelzine were better than a placebo in treatment of melancholic major depressives and dysthymics. Although Donaldson (18) had suggested that tolerance may develop to the effects of phenelzine among depressives, Harrison et al. (19) showed in a double-blind study that the acute antidepressant effects of phenelzine are probably maintained for at least 6 months. Twelve dysthymic patients showed a positive response to acute phenelzine treatment; of these twelve, all seven of those randomly assigned to continuation treatment on a placebo relapsed, but only one of five patients assigned to continuation treatment with phenelzine relapsed. Taken together, these findings suggest that phenelzine may be effective in the acute and continuing treatment of dysthymia.

   c. *Serotonergic Specific Reuptake Inhibitors.*   Only one randomized double-blind trial of an SSRI in dysthymia is readily available. Hellerstein et al. (20) studied the effectiveness of fluoxetine during a period of 8 weeks in 32 patients who met DSM-III-R criteria for dysthymia. Ten of 16 patients randomly assigned to receive fluoxetine showed treatment response (62.5%), although only three of 16 assigned to the placebo group showed a response (18.8%). An important limitation of this study is its short duration. Since dysthymia is by definition a chronic condition, it is reasonable to speculate that a larger percentage of patients would respond to longer trials. Further research on the effectiveness of SSRIs in dysthymia is clearly warranted, especially because of their more benign side-effect profile in comparison to the TCAs.

   d. *Reversible Inhibitors of Monoamine Oxidase.*   Moclobemide is the RIMA most widely studied in treatment of dysthymia. It is not currently available in the United States, but it is available in Europe, South America, and Canada. A meta-analysis presented by Angst and Stable (21) showed that moclobemide has a similar spectrum of effect in depression as do the TCAs. It is effective in patients with double depression (major depression superimposed on dysthymia), with an overall ''good'' response rate of 63%. They do not, however, report on studies of the treatment of dysthymia without concomitant major depression.

   Petursson (22) reviews studies of RIMAs in dysthymia and in dysthymic-like conditions. This author reports on several studies of moclobemide in dysthymia and finds that such studies have generally shown that moclobemide has an efficacy similar to that of TCAs and SSRIs in the treatment of dysthymia, although many studies have suffered from diagnostic uncertainty and other methodological inadequacies.

e. Ritanserin. Ritanserin is a 5-HT2 antagonist that may have antidepressant properties. Its safety and benign side-effect profile make it a potentially valuable addition to the list of available antidepressant medications. Bersani et al. (23) showed that a large percentage of dysthymic patients had a therapeutic response to this agent in a double-blind, placebo-controlled study. Bakish et al. (9) reported a double-blind, placebo-controlled comparison of ritanserin, imipramine, and placebo in outpatients with dysthymia by DSM-III criteria. They found that both imipramine and ritanserin were effective in dysthymia. There was some evidence that imipramine was more effective than ritanserin; this was balanced by evidence of imipramine's greater side-effect liability. Although not currently widely available for clinical use, ritanserin may be a potentially useful agent for the treatment of dysthymia, and study of its effectiveness in the disorder will likely continue.

f. Summary. Review of studies of the treatment of dysthymia allows several conclusions. Although in the past dysthymia was thought to be characterological and thus not amenable to pharmacological treatment, evidence accumulated over the last several decades has shown that dysthymia is probably biologically related to other mood disorders. Studies have clearly shown that most people with dysthymia respond to pharmacological treatment with TCAs, MAOIs, SSRIs, and ritanserin, even when patients present with double depression or depressive symptoms of many years' standing. Pharmacological treatment should at least be considered in any case of dysthymia; many clinicians might argue that it is indicated in most, if not all, cases.

Selection of antidepressant medication for treatment of dysthymia should be guided by the degree to which the agent has been shown effective, its side-effect profile, and its safety in recovering addicts. Safety is determined by at least three properties of the antidepressant: 1) the medication's therapeutic index (simply put, the ratio between harmful and therapeutically useful doses of the medication); 2) the extent to which it may interact with substances of abuse; and 3) the lethality of the agent in suicide attempts (24).

Lithium is a medication with a relatively narrow therapeutic index, for example. The difference between a dose of lithium that produces desirable therapeutic effects and one that produces undesirable and even harmful adverse effects is comparatively small. Although not often used alone as an antidepressant, lithium is used in the treatment of bipolar disorders (which may be comorbid with addictive disorders) and as an augmenting agent in the treatment of depression refractory to monotherapy. The consumption of alcohol by patients on lithium may potentiate its adverse effects, and its use in a recovering addict who may be prone to relapse may be inadvisable. All other antidepressants, but especially the TCAs, may interact with alcohol to increase central nervous system (CNS) depression, thus resulting in a net decrease in the therapeutic safety margin of these medications.

Perhaps the best known interaction of antidepressants with substances of abuse is that of the MAOIs and alcoholic beverages containing the amino acid tyramine. Ingestion of such beverages when a patient is taking an MAOI may result in sudden and potentially lethal increases in the patient's blood pressure. For this reason, although MAOIs are effective antidepressants, they may be a less desirable choice for the depressed alcoholic. Similarly, MAOIs may interact with cocaine, resulting in possible lethal blood pressure elevations as well. The MAOIs can also interact with meperidine, resulting in agitation, elevated body temperature, tachycardia, and hypertension.

The risk of successful suicide by overdose with TCAs is much higher than with an overdose of other antidepressants. An overdose of as little as 1,000 mg of a TCA may be lethal; inasmuch as a typical daily dose of a TCA may be 300 mg–400 mg, it may easily be seen that even a week's prescription of this class of antidepressant may be extremely hazardous in a suicidal patient. Although the TCAs are the agents most clearly shown to be effective in dysthymia treatment, their use may be limited by their safety and their side effects. The MAOIs may also be useful in dysthymia but share similar limitations with the TCAs. The overall pattern of studies suggests that the newer serotonergic agents may be effective in treatment of dysthymia, and the clinician may elect to begin treatment with one of these agents, such as fluoxetine or sertraline, and progress to other agents depending on patient response.

2. *Psychotherapy*

As with pharmacotherapy, the purpose of this section is not to exhaustively review studies on the psychotherapy of dysthymia, but rather to summarize relevant research briefly (for reviews, see [25;26]). Research on the psychotherapy of dysthymia is, in most cases, rudimentary. Studies have usually not used large numbers of patients, standardized treatment protocols, or followed up with patients for adequate periods to allow evaluation of treatment effects. In spite of these serious shortcomings, a few studies have suggested that psychotherapy has a role in the treatment of dysthymia. The two approaches best studied are cognitive-behavioral therapy (CBT) and interpersonal psychotherapy (IPT).

a.   Cognitive Behavioral Therapy.   The theoretical underpinning of CBT includes the central idea that mood symptoms result from distortions in the way in which patients perceive and interpret events around them. Patients are taught to recognize their cognitive distortions and to work actively to counteract them. A typical and clinically relevant example of this process might be the patient who experiences a minor setback in his or her personal life. If the patient were to engage in ''all or nothing'' thinking, he or she might respond to the minor setback by interpreting a minor instance as a rule. The patient might view the minor setback as an illustration that, ''I'm always a failure'' or ''I can never succeed.'' With CBT, the patient is taught to recognize this distorted pattern of thinking and to counteract it by thinking more realistically. This sort of ''all or nothing'' thinking may occur in recovering addicts striving to remain abstinent; other types of cognitive distortions may also occur in mood disordered and addicted patients. Several investigators have applied variants of this basic therapeutic approach in treating dysthymia.

Harpin et al. (27) provided cognitive therapy to six patients and compared results of twice weekly cognitive therapy with a control group of six patients placed on a waiting list. All patients were described as not having improved with use of antidepressant medication. Patients who received CBT during a period of 10 weeks showed a significant decline in scores on the Hamilton Depression Rating Scale. Several active-treatment patients continued to show gains at 6-month follow-up, whereas none of the control subjects had improved. McCullough (28) describes CBT of 10 dysthymic patients. All patients in this study improved as measured by the Beck Depression Inventory, and nine patients were described as remaining in remission 2 years later.

These results suggest the potential usefulness of CBT in dysthymia. In Markowitz' review (25), seven studies that used some form of CBT in treating dysthymic patients were reviewed. During the seven studies, 116 patients were treated, and of these, 41% improved with CBT. It is thus a promising modality for the treatment of medication-unresponsive patients and is likely an important adjunct to treatment of dysthymia with medication.

Coping skills therapy is a variant of CBT developed specifically for the treatment of alcoholism. It has also been adapted for the treatment of cocaine dependence. This approach focuses on identifying those factors likely to trigger relapse in the recovering addict and helps him or her develop ways to avoid or cope with these triggers without addictive behavior. Alcoholic patients who sampled alcohol while undergoing treatment with coping skills therapy and naltrexone had a lower relapse rate than those treated with naltrexone and supportive therapy (29), suggesting that this therapy may be useful with other addicted and depressed patients. Elements of CBT for depression could be combined with coping skills therapy to obtain optimal response in dysthymic patients with addictive disorders.

b. Interpersonal Psychotherapy.   IPT is based on the premise that intense affective experiences are mainly interpersonal and that disruptions in important interpersonal relations are causally related to mood disorders. This time-limited treatment focuses on diagnosis and resolution of interpersonal relations difficulties that fall into several major categories, such as unresolved grief, social role conflicts, or social skills deficits.

Markowitz (25) reports that his group at Cornell University developed a manual for IPT with dysthymics. At present, only limited data are available on its effectiveness. In a study reported by Mason et al. (30), nine dysthymic patients were treated. Five of these patients had not responded to adequate doses of desipramine, and four had declined treatment with medication. These patients received an average of 12 sessions of IPT and showed substantial decreases in their scores on the Hamilton Depression Rating Scale. In a separate study, the use of IPT with HIV-positive men was investigated (31). Two men with dysthymia were included in this study. Both showed substantial improvement in their dysthymic symptoms with either 12 or 16 sessions of IPT, as measured by change in the scores on the Hamilton Rating Scale.

Markowitz (25) further reports results of a pilot study of IPT with dysthymics. Six dysthymic patients were treated and most showed substantial changes in their report of depressive symptoms as measured by the Beck Depression Inventory. Markowitz further notes that patients responding to IPT are seen for monthly continuation sessions and most have maintained their improvement over time.

c. Summary. Only preliminary conclusions can be drawn about the usefulness of psychotherapy with dysthymics. From results such as those reviewed above, it is likely that at least some patients with dysthymia will respond to psychotherapy alone. It is especially noteworthy that some patients with poor response to medication may respond to psychotherapy. Failure of adequate trials of antidepressant medications may be an indication for psychotherapy, if it has not already been provided. It is also noteworthy that several of the CBT treatments discussed above, as well as the more routine IPT, focused treatment efforts on interpersonal relations difficulties. An emphasis on interpersonal relations difficulties may, therefore, be a desirable goal in psychotherapy with dysthymics; this may be doubly true in psychotherapy of the recovering addict with dysthymia.

C. Summary

This chapter has briefly reviewed the evidence for dysthymia as a distinct mood disorder that may be related to other mood disorders. Although the overlap between dysthymia and addictions is unclear, the clinician working with recovering addicts will likely see some patients with dysthymia. Understanding the nature and treatability of the disorder is important, because dysthymia is a demonstrated risk factor for the development of major depression and could well be a factor in relapse to addiction. Several types of medication, including TCAs, MAOIs, SSRIs, and ritanserin, may be effective in treating dysthymia. Although studies of psychotherapy with dysthymics are methodologically limited, the data that are available show that psychotherapy alone may be an effective treatment. This is particularly important to note, because some patients will either fail to respond to medication or choose not to undergo treatment with medication. An important but unanswered question is the extent to which psychotherapy and pharmacotherapy may be complementary or even synergistic in acute dysthymia treatment. The role of psychotherapy in preventing relapse of mood symptoms is unknown, but it clearly has practical importance. Finally, although it has been shown that antidepressants may be valuable adjuncts in the treatment of some addictions, notably alcoholism, the complex relation of mood symptoms, addictive behavior, and antidepressant treatment requires further elucidation.

REFERENCES

1. H. S. Akiskal, Dysthymia: Clinical and External Validity, *Acta Psychiatr. Scand., 89*(suppl 383):19–23 (1994).
2. American Psychiatric Association: *Diagnostic and Statistical Manual, 4th ed.,* American Psychiatric Press, Washington, D.C., 1994a, p. 345.
3. American Psychiatric Association: *Diagnostic and Statistical Manual, 4th ed.,* American Psychiatric Press, Washington, DC, 1994b, pp. 345–346.
4. American Psychiatric Association: *Diagnostic and Statistical Manual, 4th ed.,* American Psychiatric Press, Washington, DC, 1994c, p. 718.
5. American Psychiatric Association: *Diagnostic and Statistical Manual, 4th ed.,* American Psychiatric Press, Washington, DC, 1994d, pp. 732–733.
6. J. H. Kocsis, A. J. Frances, C. Voss, J. Mann, B. J. Mason, and J. Sweeney, Imipramine Treatment for Chronic Depression, *Arch. Gen. Psychiatry 45:*253–257 (1988a).
7. J. H. Kocsis, A. J. Frances, C. Voss, B. J. Mason, J. Mann, and J. Sweeney, Imipramine and Social-Vocational Adjustment in Chronic Depression, *Am. J. Psychiatry 145:*997–999 (1988b).
8. J. H. Kocsis, B. J. Mason, A. J. Frances, J. Sweeney, J. J. Mann, and D. Marin, Prediction of Response of Chronic Depression to Imipramine, *J. Affective Disord. 17:*255–260 (1989).
9. D. Bakish, Y. D. Lapierre, R. Weinstein, J. Klein, A. Wiens et al., Ritanserin, Imipramine, and Placebo in the Treatment of Dysthymic Disorder, *J. Clin. Psychopharmacol. 13:*409–414 (1993).
10. D. B. Marin, J. H. Kocsis, A. J. Frances, and M. Parides, Desipramine

for the Treatment of "Pure" Dysthymia versus "Double" Depression, *Am. J. Psychiatry 151:*1079–1080 (1994).

11. A. Kornhaber and I. M. Horwitz, A Comparison of Clomipramine and Doxepin in Neurotic Depression, *J. Clin. Psychiatry 45:*337–341 (1984).

12. E. S. Paykel, P. R. Rowan, R. R. Parker, and A. V. Bhat, Response to Phenelzine and Amitriptyline in Subtypes of Outpatient Depression, *Arch. Gen. Psychiatry 39:*1041–1049 (1982).

13. E. V. Nunes, P. J. McGrath, F. M. Quitkin, J. P. Stewart, W. Harrison, et al., Imipramine Treatment of Alcoholism with Comorbid Depression, *Am. J. Psychiatry 150:*963–965 (1993).

14. B. J. Mason and J. H. Kocsis, Desipramine Treatment of Alcoholism, *Psychopharmacol. Bulletin 27:*155–161 (1991).

15. R. L. Ownby and P. J. Goodnick, Predictors of Response to the Monoamine Oxidase Inhibitors, In:*Predictors of Treatment Response in Mood Disorders* (P. J. Goodnick, ed.), American Psychiatric Press, Washington, D.C., 1995.

16. J. W. Stewart, F. M. Quitkin, P. J. McGrath et al., Social Functioning in Chronic Depression: 6 Weeks of Antidepressant Treatment. *Psychiatry Res. 25:*213–222 (1988).

17. J. Vallejo, C. Gasto, R. Catalan et al., Double-Blind Study of Imipramine versus Phenelzine in Melancholic and Dysthymic Disorders, *Br. J. Psychiatry 151:*639–642 (1987).

18. S. R. Donaldson, Tolerance to Phenelzine and Subsequent Refractory Depression: Three Cases, *J. Clin. Psychiatry 50:*33–35 (1989).

19. W. Harrison, J. Rabkin, J. W. Stewart, P. J. McGrath, E. Tricamo, and F. Quitkin, Phenelzine for Chronic Depression: A Study of Continuation Treatment, *J. Clin. Psychiatry 47:*346–349 (1986).

20. D. J. Hellerstein, P. Yanowitch, J. Rosenthal, L. W. Samstag, M. Maurer M, et al., A Randomized Double-Blind Study of Fluoxetine versus Placebo in the Treatment of Dysthymia, *Am. J. Psychiatry 150:*1169–1175 (1993).

21. J. Angst and M. Stabl, Efficacy of Moclobemide in Different Patients Groups: A Meta-Analysis of Studies, *Psychopharmacology 106:*S109–S113 (1992).

22. H. Petursson, Studies of Reversible and Selective Inhibitors of Monoamine Oxidase A in Dysthymia, *Acta Psychiatr. Scand. 91*(suppl 386): 36–39 (1995).

23. G. Bersani, F. Pozzi, S. Marini, A. Grisoini, A. Pasini, and N. Ciani, 5HT2 Receptor Antagonism in Dysthymic Disorder: A Double-Blind Placebo Control with Ritanserin, *Acta Psychiatr. Scand. 83:*244–248 (1991).

24. P. G. Janicak, J. M. Davis, S. H. Preskorn, and F. J. Ayd, *Principles and Practice of Psychopharmacotherapy*, Williams & Wilkins, Baltimore 1993, pp. 278–279.

25. J. C. Markowitz, Psychotherapy of Dysthymia, *Am. J. Psychiatry 151*:1114–1121 (1994).

26. E. S. Paykel, Psychological Therapies, *Acta Psychiatr. Scand., 89*(Suppl 383):35–41 (1994).

27. R. E. Harpin, R. P. Liberman RP, I. Marks, R. Stern, and W. E. Bohanno, Cognitive-Behavioral Therapy for Chronically Depressed Patients: A Controlled Pilot Study, *J. Nerv. Ment. Dis. 170*:295–301 (1982).

28. J. P. McCullough, Psychotherapy for Dysthymia: A Naturalistic Study of Ten Patients, *J. Nerv. Ment. Dis. 179*:734–740 (1991).

29. S. S. O'Malley, A. J. Jaffe, G. Chang, R. S. Schottenfeld, R. E. Meyer, and B. Rounsaville, Naltrexone and Coping Skills Therapy for Alcohol Dependence. *Arch. Gen. Psychiatry 49*:881–887 (1992).

30. B. J. Mason, J. C. Markowitz, and G. L. Klerman, IPT for Dysthymic Disorders, In: *New Applications of Interpersonal Psychotherapy* (G. L. Klerman, and M. M. Weissman, eds.), American Psychiatric Press, Washington, D.C., 1993.

31. J. C. Markowitz, G. L. Klerman, S. Perry, Interpersonal Psychotherapy of Depressed HIV-Seropositive Outpatients. *Hosp. Community Psychiatry 43*:885–890 (1992).

6

Treatment of Bipolar Disorders

Mary J. Kujawa and Joseph R. Calabrese
University Hospitals of Cleveland and Case Western Reserve University School of Medicine, Cleveland, Ohio

I. INTRODUCTION

The relationship between alcohol and drug abuse and mood disorders has long been postulated; it was Plato who first referred to the potential of alcohol to cause symptoms suggestive of mania (1). Several centuries later, Kraepelin (2) noted that some episodes of mania occasionally present as delirium tremens. More recently LSD- and PCP-induced manic attacks have been observed in biologically vulnerable individuals. Substance abuse comorbidity is observed to occur in more than half of all patients with bipolar disorder. The Epidemiologic Catchment Area (ECA) study demonstrated that more than 50% of treated substance-abuse patients had a dual diagnosis, and a large proportion of these had bipolar illness (3). It is clear that comorbidity for bipolar illness and substance abuse has a notable impact on morbidity and mortality; suicide and outcome measures such as relapse rate, recidivism in rehabilitation, natural history of the illness, and prognosis, are all affected.

What remains less clear is the relative contribution of each, or even which is primary in impact. For example, suicide, homicide, aggression, and impulsivity, frequently associated with alcoholism and alcohol intoxication, are also associated with bipolar illness. Other confounding variables include:

(a) alcohol/sedatives can cause depressive symptoms;
(b) signs of temporary, but severe, depressive symptoms can follow prolonged alcohol/sedative abuse;
(c) alcohol/sedative abuse can escalate during affective episodes, especially mania;
(d) depressive symptoms and alcohol/sedative abuse occur in other psychiatric disorders;
(e) many bipolar patients have independent alcoholism or substance abuse disorders; and
(f) it remains unclear why and to what extent bipolar patients self-administer alcohol and drugs for relief of affective symptoms.

Effective treatment requires accurate psychiatric diagnosis and evaluation of the impact of substance abuse over time. Specific and early treatment of the underlying psychiatric diagnosis may result in a decrease in the morbidity and mortality of these patients, including restoration of a euthymic state, retention in treatment, and prevention of relapse. In this chapter, we will review the phenomenologic interface between substance abuse and bipolar disorder, the clinical management of these patients, prevalence rates, and some methodological issues limiting the currently available studies.

II. PHENOMENOLOGY

The phenomenology of individual disease states alone and their patterns of coexistence affect not only their presentation but also prognosis and treatment response. Using operational criteria for cyclothymia, Akiskal and coworkers (4) suggested that these patients resort to alcohol and drug abuse as a means of self-treatment or augmenting excitement. Fifty percent of patients with cyclothymia exhibited drug and alcohol abuse (5). When bipolar patients engage in sedative or stimulant abuse in an attempt to self-treat refractory illness or enhance symptoms of the bipolar illness, special consideration must be given in treatment. Substance abuse through self-medication to alleviate or intensify affective symptoms clearly occurs. The clinician also must not overlook the possibility that drug or alcohol abuse is precipitating underlying bipolar illness and modifying the course and expression of bipolar illness in patients who abuse substances. The latter appears to be especially true in those who have mixed states or who are rapid cyclers (6, 7).

Discerning whether substance abuse is primary or secondary in bipolar patients is often problematic. Factors that have been shown to be helpful include chronology of symptom presentation, severity of presenting symptoms, family history (8, 9), and age (10). An increased prevalence of alcoholism in relatives of male bipolar probands has been noted (11). Results from other studies, however, have not been consistent. Dunner and coworkers (12) found no greater rate of alcoholism in families of bipolar I or unipolar depression probands when compared with control families. The rate of alcoholism was found to be increased in the families of bipolar II probands, however. Morrison (13) found no increased rate of alcoholism in families of bipolar patients, unless the patients themselves were alcoholics. Those abusing alcohol before the age of 20 have been found to be more likely to exhibit hostility, physical violence, depression, and to attempt suicide than older-onset alcoholics (10). This was also reflected in the ECA study (3), which showed that much of the overlap of mood disorders with alcoholism comes with type II alcoholics. These early onset, impulsive, antisocial, thrill-seeking alcoholics exhibit a 6%–9% prevalence rate of bipolar disorder. Alcoholism, depression, bipolar illness, and antisocial personality all appear to have a strong genetic predisposition; they sometimes run in the same families and may appear in the same individual. Many studies suggest these are separate, etiologically and clinically, and are not alternative manifestations of the same underlying disease process (14). Others, however, have argued a common connection with low cerebrospinal fluid (CSF) 5-HIAA (15). Although controversy remains, the clinical consensus is that the most clinically consistent predictors of primary emphasis remain chronology and severity of presenting symptoms.

There is a common assumption that substance abuse in bipolar I patients is largely state dependent and only occurs during the symptomatic interval. This was challenged by the ECA study, which showed a predominance of persistent dependence over abuse in this population. Of bipolar I patients, 15% exhibited alcohol abuse, compared with 31% who were alcohol dependent. Likewise, drug dependence (28%) was more common than drug abuse (13%) in this patient population. Bipolar II patients are also more likely to show chronic abuse patterns. The ECA study was not designed to evaluate the phenomenon of self treatment.

III. CLINICAL MANAGEMENT

Given the lack of adequate data in the literature and the persistence of controversy, it is difficult to provide uniform treatment recommendations for patients who experience symptoms suggestive of both substance abuse and bipolar disorders. However, some general considerations for the management of patients with this kind of comorbidity follow.

In the experience of the authors, differential diagnoses that labor over whether a patient has primary bipolar disorder with secondary substance abuse or primary substance abuse disorder with secondary symptoms of bipolar disorder do not appear to be useful. More often than not, patients require simultaneous treatment for both entities, regardless of what is secondary and what is primary. Perhaps the most conservative therapeutic posture is to assume that patients have both illnesses and to develop a care plan that addresses the needs of both. After implementing the care plan, one can modify the specific treatment modalities used in the care plan as the relative importance of the different symptoms becomes evident. This approach, however, could be faulted for leading to overtreatment, increased cost, the potential for noncompliance, and development of unnecessary side effects. Given the fact that the likelihood for relapse with each of these disorders is high, pursuing a more aggressive treatment plan appears prudent.

Basing treatment on the chronology of presenting symptoms, severity of presenting symptoms, and family history are all very helpful in developing well-rounded care plans. The importance of a detailed chronology of the onset of symptoms is often critical to successful treatment. For example, did the difficulties with affective symptoms predate substance abuse? If this is the case, treating the mood disorder will, in some instances, also resolve or mitigate the substance abuse problem. The presence of another mental illness is an important factor in relapse prevention for substance abuse and dependence disorders. There is some evidence that suggests that treatment matching based on psychiatric severity improves outcome (16, 17).

When substance abuse is entirely state dependent, it often remits spontaneously when the mood disorder is successfully treated. However, when substance abuse occurs predominantly during the euthymic interval, prognosis is markedly affected, and formal involvement in a 12-step group is always indicated.

Patients who present with both substance abuse and bipolar disorders require treatment with pharmacotherapy and counseling. Medication management should be designed to prevent a recurrence of major mood swings, whereas counseling should be directed toward the need for illness education and complete abstinence. The psychoeducation treatment model is especially useful for patients with these illnesses because of the confusion that usually occurs regarding issues of symptom causality, diagnosis, treatment, and prognosis.

Patients who present with mixed states and bipolar II disorder are at increased risk of substance abuse; they are, therefore, more likely to be unresponsive to the mood stabilizing properties of lithium. These patients usually require treatment with an anticonvulsant, either valproate or carbamazepine. The presence of alcohol abuse is associated with diminished lithium response in the control of mania (6). It is unclear whether this response is the result of poor compliance with lithium therapy or diminished effectiveness of the drug. Alcohol abuse may be more strongly associated with mixed states that result from a relatively poor prophylactic response to lithium. It is clear that poor prophylactic response to lithium has been correlated to the coexistence of drug abuse (18).

There is some emerging evidence to suggest that mood stabilizers might also have efficacy in the treatment of drug-related withdrawal symptoms. The antikindling effects of carbamazepine may prove useful in the treatment of patients with prolonged cocaine cravings or cocaine-induced paranoia (19). Preclinical data supports the efficacy of both carbamazepine and valproate in alcohol, and possibly benzodiazepine, withdrawal.

A. Pharmacotherapy

The medication algorithm in Figure 1 is designed to assist the clinician in the medical management of bipolar disorder. The algorithm displays a pharmacotherapy routine that is directed toward the need for long-term prophylaxis and does not emphasize acute management with unimodal agents such as a benzodiazepine, a typical antipsychotic agent, or one of the antidepressants. The algorithm attempts to assimilate the consensus of clinical opinion with the currently available drug trial data.

Starting with the first line, every other line in this algorithm describes a treatment intervention and is framed by squares or rectangles. Starting with the second line, every other line in the algorithm describes a response to a treatment intervention and is framed by circles. The first tier in this algorithm includes the first-line mood stabilizers: lithium, divalproex sodium, and carbamazepine. Only 60% to 80% of patients respond to lithium; the following are predictors of lithium nonresponse: mixed hypomanias/manias, rapid cycling, continuous circular cycling, patterns in which mania is preceded by depression and followed by euthymia, mood incongruent psychotic symptoms, bipolar type II presentations, negative family histories, and presentations comorbid with substance abuse or borderline personality. Alcohol and substance abuse may, in fact, be the most common predictors of lithium nonresponse because more than half of bipolar patients demonstrate comorbidity. Although many psychiatrists still consider lithium to be the treatment of choice for bipolar disorder of all types, there is growing opinion that patients with either mixed manias or rapid cycling patients should be treated with an anticonvulsant medication before lithium is started.

The second tier in this algorithm includes augmentation with one of the alternative agents not previously used in tier one. This augmentation paradigm is recommended for both partial responders and complete nonresponders. The recommendation in the second tier is that even in the absence of any response, the original agent should be continued

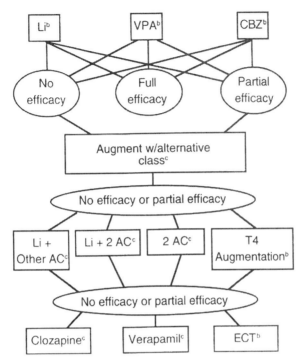

Figure 1 Psychopharmacology algorithm. AHCPR strength of evidence codes: a, good research-based evidence—some opinion; b, fair research-based evidence—substantial opinion; c, poor research-based evidence—primarily opinion.

and then augmented. This recommendation is predicted on the assumption that it may take more than one cycle length for a given prophylactic treatment to become expressed, particularly in the presence of long-standing, circular, continuous rapid cycling.

The third tier in this algorithm includes an array of recommendations that are controversial. The first option is to continue lithium therapy while replacing one anticonvulsant with another. This recommendation is based on case report data that indicate that nonresponse to one anticonvulsant does not predict nonresponse to another. A second option allows for the addition of a third mood stabilizer to the regimen of the first two, i.e., treating with lithium, divalproex, and carbamazepine all at the same time. However, if it is clear that the lithium did not result in even a partial initial response, the more prudent consideration would be to discontinue lithium and replace it with a second anticonvulsant. This recommendation is predicated on the assumption that anticonvulsant efficacy is additive. The clinician may also supplement any combination of lithium, divalproex, or carbamazepine with a thyroid preparation, usually tetraiodothyronine (T4).

The fourth tier in this algorithm includes interventions that are clearly either controversial or complicated. These include the use of electroconvulsive therapy, clozapine, and such calcium channel blockers as verapamil and nimodipine.

As a result of inadequately controlled data in the classic bipolar literature, there is substantial controversy regarding pharmacotherapy for the management of break-through manias and severe depressions. Throughout each tier in the algorithm, it is assumed that one or more of the benzodiazepines or typical antipsychotic agents may be prescribed to treat break-through symptoms, but they would not be used as primary maintenance therapies. However, special precautions must be taken when using a benzodiazepine for the acute nonspecific management of mania; these agents should probably be avoided entirely in bipolar II patients who have a history of sedative or alcohol abuse.

The convention regarding the management of depression is more complex and more controversial. Recent data suggest that monoamine oxidase inhibitors are more effective antidepressants than the tricyclic antidepressants for treating classic bipolar depressions (20).

IV. PREVALENCE RATES

During the last 10 years, substantial controversy has emerged over issues regarding the primary vs. secondary nature of diagnostic cormorbidity. Frequently, it is falsely assumed that secondary cormorbidity spontaneously remits when the primary source of psychopathology is effectively treated. This controversy is particularly relevant to the interface between substance abuse and bipolar disorders, because there is substantial syndromal overlap between these two categories of illnesses; both involve disturbances of mood and affect (21). When mood disorders coexist with substance abuse disorders, it is often difficult to ascertain which is primary. With the advent of health care reform through managed care, providers are being pressured to use the most efficient form of treatment for the shortest period of time. Substantial amounts of time are invested in this exercise of differential diagnosis, and there is emerging consensus that the best outcomes are obtained by treating both disorders simultaneously when diagnostic criteria for both are met.

Past studies of prevalence rates were compromised either by the absence of uniform diagnostic criteria or by the use of different nomenclatures. These differences had substantial impact on the estimation of comorbidity prevalence rates (22). More recent studies have uniformly used either the Diagnostic and Statistical Manual of Mental Disorders (third version, 1978) (DSM-III-R), its revised version which was released in 1987, or the Research Diagnostic Criteria (RDC). With the arrival of the DSM-III, the diagnostic criteria for substance abuse became more stringent, and it was this nomenclature that was used in the ECA study (3). This pivotal study has gained much attention, because it is the largest population-based assessment of comorbidity to date.

Heterogeneity among bipolar patients is common; it has clouded interpretation of research results and compromised the ability of the clinician to develop effective and efficient care plans. Recent changes in the DSM-IV provide the clinician with better tools to describe different clinically significant patterns of presentation. These specifiers, which include rapid cycling, have been determined to have substantial impact on course, prognosis, and comorbidity.

The essential feature of bipolar I disorder is one or more manic episodes, usually accompanied by one or more major depressive episodes. The minimum duration criteria is 14 days for depression and 7 days for mania. Bipolar II disorder consists of at least one hypomanic episode and at least one major depressive episode. The minimum duration criteria for depression is again 14 days, but only 4 days for hypomania. Since the DSM-III-R did not use any minimum duration criteria for mania or hypomania, this additional rigor may impact on the rate at which this illness is diagnosed by clinicians.

Cyclothymic disorder refers to the presence of numerous hypomanic episodes and numerous periods of depressed mood or loss of interest or pleasure that do not meet criteria for major depression for at least 2 years. Rapid cycling has been used to specify courses that include four or more episodes of depression, mania, or hypomania in the previous 12 months. Patients do not have to sustain a euthymic interval between a mania and a depression for these to be counted as two episodes. Numbers of episodes are tabulated, rather than numbers of cycles. For example, two cycles in which manic episodes are biphasically coupled with depressions followed by euthymic intervals would count as four episodes and satisfy criteria for rapid cycling.

Episodes are demarcated by a switch to an episode of opposite polarity or by a period of remission. The DSM-IV notes that organic factors may induce mania and divides them into substance induced (categorized under substance use disorders) and those not induced by substance (categorized under organic affective syndromes). Affective episodes induced by substance abuse, however, are not counted.

Drugs thought to cause mania and hypomania include phencyclidine, the hallucinogens, alcohol, barbiturates, and benzodiazepines. Mixed states have been especially vulnerable to the inadequacies of diagnostic systems; they have been considered as transitional from one phase of illness to another and as independent clinical states combining mixtures of mood, thought, and activity components.

A. Rate of Substance Abuse in Primary Mood Disorders

The rates of alcohol abuse and alcoholism in patients with bipolar illness range from 3%–75%; the range in the general population is 2.6%–15.7% (23–28). However, when bipolar patients are questioned specifically about their alcohol use, 60%–75% report increased consumption (23, 29, 30). The ECA data indicate that during a patient's lifetime, alcohol abuse or dependence and bipolar I disorder coexist at a rate of 46%. Although mania was shown to be strongly associated with alcoholism (odds ratio = 6.2), this was not the case for recurrent major depression (odds ratio = 1.7) (3). The rates at which bipolar disorder and drug abuse coexist are somewhat less than those of alcohol abuse. In the ECA study, the rate of drug abuse or dependence in bipolar I disorder was 41% as compared to 18% in recurrent major depression.

The rate of cocaine abuse in bipolar patients is substantially higher than in the general population (27, 28). In contrast to what a clinician might expect, the majority of bipolar patients who use cocaine do so more often when manic than when depressed. Esteroff and coworkers reported that 58% of bipolar patients in the manic phase of the illness abused cocaine, whereas only 30% of those in the depressed phase did so (30). From the ECA study, the odds ratio that a cocaine abuser will have bipolar I disorder is 11. For example, a patient with bipolar I disorder is 11 times more likely to abuse cocaine than someone in the general population. The odds ratio that a cocaine abuser will have bipolar II disorder is 20; the odds ratio that a cocaine abuser will have recurrent major depression is 3 (3). These data indicate that the formal entry of bipolar II disorder into our DSM-IV nomenclature is of particular relevance to the clinician. Substance abuse is much more common in bipolar II disorder, and presentations involving this kind of cormorbidity are commonly seen. The overall rate of bipolar affective disorder was higher among chronic cocaine abusers than any other type of drug abusers (31).

The rates of recurrent major depression are more evenly distributed across the different types of drug abuse (32). It is unclear which bipolar symptoms are secondary to drug abuse, or whether other features of bipolar disorder lead to greater cocaine abuse. In addition to differences in substance abuse rates between bipolar I and II disorders, there is also evidence to suggest a gender difference. Women with bipolar II disorder are much more likely to abuse alcohol than those with bipolar I (12% vs. 0%). In contrast, there is little impact of subtype for males (type I, 19% vs. type II, 21%) (33, 34). In another study, it was noted that women with bipolar II disorder had higher rates of alcoholism than those with bipolar I disorder or unipolar major depression (35).

Bipolar patients with mixed states account for about 40% of all patients, and as many as 60%–70% exhibit poor response to lithium. Kraepelin is credited for having first considered the clinical importance of mixed states. He noted, ''. . . we meet temporarily with states which do not exactly correspond to manic excitement or to depression, but represent a mixture of morbid symptoms of both forms of manic-depressive insanity.'' Mixed states may appear as a transitional phenomenon in an otherwise classic bipolar course, or they may appear independently and dominate the clinical picture. Mixed states imply a variant of bipolar disorder that is more likely to become chronic, recurrent, comorbid with substance abuse and symptomatology, lithium nonresponsive; it is also likely to respond to anticonvulsants. Substance abuse is common in patients with cyclothymic disorder; the clinical impression is that many of these patients use substances as a form of self-treatment. Typically, sedatives and alcohol are used during depressed periods and stimulants and psychedelic substances during hypomanic periods (36).

B. Rate of Mood Disorders in Primary Substance Abuse Disorders

The lack of consistency in diagnostic criteria has led to widely disparate estimates of the rate of depression in alcoholism, ranging from 3%–98% (37, 38). When semistructured, semistandardized research diagnostic interviews are used to look for the coexistence of mood disorders in patients with primary alcoholism, 12%–57% will show this kind of comorbidity. However, when observer-rated depression scales are used to ascertain the presence of subsyndromal depressive symptoms, the prevalence of this kind of comorbidity increases to as high as 98% (39).

It is clear that there is a significantly higher rate of mood disorders among alcoholics as compared to the general population. In particular, the prevalence rate of bipolar disorder in a population of alcoholics is 6%–9% (26, 40–43). This is three to four times greater than that seen in the general population (1%–2%) (26). The rate of primary mood disorders with alcohol abuse ranges from 6%–46%, compared with secondary affective disorder and alcohol abuse rates of 24%–41%. There do not appear to be differences among bipolar, recurrent major depression, dysthymic, or cyclothymic disorders.

V. METHODOLOGIC ISSUES

The rigor of the scientific literature evaluating the phenomenology of bipolar disorder and its treatment is seriously encumbered by the three mood states that accompany this illness and its multiple patterns of presentation. Studies involving the rapid cycling pattern of bipolar disorders, as well as presentations with mixed hypomanic/manic states are particularly challenging. Due to the illness's inherent complexity, the broad spectrum of bipolar disorder research has been viewed as labor-intensive and expensive. This is particularly the case in studies that attempt to evaluate issues of treatment and prognosis in patients who have both substance abuse and bipolar disorders. Many studies have not used semi-structured, semistandardized diagnostic research interviews, and some have made diagnoses without the benefit of standardized criteria, either the DSM or the RDC. Using rating scales to determine the severity of affective symptoms in patients diagnosed by a research interview is an effective way of quantifying episode severity, but using these rating scales to diagnose exaggerates prevalence rates, because secondary depressive symptoms are commonly seen in substance abuse patients with no mood disorders.

Many studies do not distinguish abuse from dependence. Frequently, there is no control group. For example, when looking at the rate at which alcoholism and depression coexist, comparisons with the general population are necessary. Another issue to consider is that bipolar disorder has a low baseline rate in the general population, and often, its relationship to alcohol and drug abuse is difficult to demonstrate, especially in small studies. In addition to the above, there are many substances that can be abused by patients, and these appear to interact differently according to gender and the different mood disorders. It is also well recognized that both substance abusing patients and patients in the hypomanic/manic phase of bipolar disorder underestimate and minimize impairment from their illnesses. For this reason, it can be particularly challenging to distinguish hypomanic elation from that of euphorigenic drugs of abuse. There is also the possibility that clinicians inadvertently underestimate the prevalence of substance abuse in patients with serious mental illnesses such as bipolar disorder and schizophrenia by focusing primarily on more emergent dramatic psychotic symptoms. In addition to the above, it is very difficult to get good information about alcohol and drug abuse in patients who are currently in the manic phase of bipolar disorder.

REFERENCES

1. E. H. Ackerknecht, *A Short History of Psychiatry,* Hafner Publishing Co., New York, 1959.
2. E. Kraepelin, *Manic Depressive Insanity and Paranoia* (G. M. Robertson, ed., translated by R. M. Barclay), E & S Livingstone, Edinburgh (1921). Reprinted Arno Press, New York, 1976.
3. D. A. Regier, M. E. Farmer, D. S. Rae, B. Z. Locke, S. J. Keith, L. L. Judd, and F. K. Goodwin, *JAMA 264:*2511 (1990).
4. H. S. Akiskal, M. K. Khani, and A. Scott-Strauss, *Psychiatr. Clin. North Am. 2:*527 (1979).
5. H. S. Akiskal, A. H. Djenderedjian, R. H. Rosenthal, and M. K. Khani, *Am. J. Psychiatry 134:*1227 (1977).
6. J. M. Himmelhoch, D. Mulla, J. F. Neil, T. P. Detre, and D. J. Kupfer, *Arch. Gen. Psychiatry 33:*1062 (1976).
7. J. M. Himmelhoch, *Psychiatr. Clin. North Am. 2:*449 (1979).
8. M. N. Hesselbrock, R. E. Meyer, and J. J. Keener, *Arch. Gen. Psychiatry 42:*1050 (1985).
9. M. A. Schuckit, *Am. J. Psychiatry 143:*140 (1986).
10. L. Buydens-Branchey, M. H. Branchey, and D. Noumair, *Arch. Gen. Psychiatry 46:*225 (1989).
11. J. E. Helzer and G. Winokur, *Arch. Gen. Psychiatry 31:*73 (1974).
12. D. L. Dunner, E. S. Gershon, and F. K. Goodwin, *Biol. Psychiatry 11:*31 (1976).
13. J. R. Morrison, *J. Nerv. Ment. Dis. 160:*227 (1975).
14. C. R. Cloninger, *Arch. Gen. Psychiatry 38:*861 (1981).
15. V. M. I. Linnoila, *J. Clin. Psychiatry 53:*46 (1992).
16. A. T. McLellan, L. Lubovsky, G. E. Woody, C. P. O'Brien, and K. A. Druley, *Arch. Gen. Psychiatry 40:*620 (1983).
17. W. Miller and R. Hester, *Treating Addictive Behaviors: Processes of Change* (W. Miller and R. Hester, ed.), Plenum Press, New York, 1986.
18. J. M. Himmelhoch, J. F. Neil, S. J. May, C. Z. Fuchs, and S. M. Licata, *Am. J. Psychiatry 137:*941 (1980).
19. J. A. Halikas, R. D. Crosby, G. A. Carlson, F. Crea, N. M. Graves, and L. D. Bowers, *Clin. Pharmacol. Ther. 50:*81 (1991).
20. J. M. Himmelhoch, M. E. Thase, A. G. Mallinger, P. Houck, *Am. J. Psychiatry 148:*910 (1991).
21. S. C. Dilsaver, *J. Clin. Psychopharm. 7:*1 (1987).
22. J. H. Boyd, M. M. Weissman, W. D. Thompson, and J. K. Myers, *Am. J. Psychiatry 140:*1309 (1983).

23. E. X. Freed, *Psychol. Rep. 25,:*280 (1969).
24. C. E. Lewis, J. Helzer, C. R. Cloninger, J. Croughan, and B. Y. Whitman, *Compr. Psychiatry 23:*451 (1982).
25. T. W. Estroff, C. A. Dackis, M. S. Gold, and A. L. C. Pottash, *Int. J. Psychiatry Med. 15:*37 (1985).
26. M. M. Weissman and J. K. Myers, *Am. J. Psychiatry 137:*372 (1980).
27. L. N. Robins, J. E. Helzer, M. M. Weissman, H. Orvaschel, E. Gruenberg, J. D. Burke, Jr., and D. A. Regier, *Arch. Gen. Psychiatry 41:*949 (1984).
28. D. A. Regier, J. H. Boyd, J. D. Burke, Jr., D. S. Rae, J. K. Myers, M. Kramer, L. N. Robins, L. K. George, M. Karno, and B. Z. Locke, *Arch. Gen. Psychiatry 45:*977 (1988).
29. J. R. Morrison, *Am. J. Psychiatry 131:*1130 (1974).
30. T. W. Estroff, C. A. Dackis, M. S. Gold, and A. L. C. Pottash, *Int. J. Psychiatry Med. 15:*37 (1985).
31. R. D. Weiss, S. M. Mirin, J. L. Michael, and A. C. Sollogub, *Am. J. Drug Alcohol Abuse 12,*17 (1986).
32. R. D. Weiss, S. M. Mirin, M. L. Griffin, and J. L. Michael, *J. Nerv. Ment. Dis. 176:*719 (1988).
33. B. Hensel, D. L. Dunner, and R. R. Fieve, *J. Affect. Disord. 1:*105 (1979).
34. D. L. Dunner, B. M. Hensel, and R. R. Fieve, *Am. J. Psychiatry 136:*583 (1979).
35. J. Endicott, J. Nee, N. Andreasen, P. Clayton, M. Keller, and W. Coryell, *J. Affective Disord. 8,*17 (1985).
36. R. D. Weiss and S. M. Mirin, *Psychiatr. Med. 3:*357 (1987).
37. M. H. Keeler, C. I. Taylor, and W. C. Miller, *Am. J. Psychiatry 136:*586 (1979).
38. J. M. Himmelhoch, S. Hill, B. Steinberg, and S. May, *J. Psychiatr. Treat. Eval. 5:*83 (1983).
39. M. W. Bernadt and R. M. Murray, *Br. J. Psychiat. 148:*393 (1986).
40. K. J. Tillotson and R. Fleming, *N. Engl. J. Med. 217:*611 (1937).
41. C. Amark, *Acta Psychiatria Neurolog. Suppl 70:*1 (1951).
42. M. J. Sherfey, *Etiology of Chronic Alcoholism* (O. Diethelm, ed.), Charles C. Thomas, Springfield, IL, 1955, p. 16.
43. R. C. Bowen, D. Cipywnyk, C. D'Arcy, and D. L. Keegan, *Can. Med. Assoc. J. 130:*869 (1984).

7

Treatment of Organic Mood Disorders

Michael Hollomon, Patricia Isbell, Mark Fulton, and Frederick Petty

Dallas Veterans Affairs Medical Center and University of Texas Southwestern Medical School, Dallas, Texas

I. INTRODUCTION

Substances of abuse alter mood. In fact, the three major substances of abuse with which this chapter deals—alcohol, cocaine, and heroin—are consumed initially for their mood altering characteristics. Eventually an addiction develops, and the substance may then be used to prevent withdrawal symptoms. In understanding the clinical presentation of patients during the process of addiction and recovery, it is important to realize that the pharmacological effects of the drugs themselves will vary, depending on the dose and physiological status of the drug user. When a drug-naive individual uses alcohol, cocaine, or heroin at low doses, the usual reaction or effect is a distinct period of pleasure or euphoria. Otherwise, there would be little reinforcement for continued use.

Once a person has developed a physiological addiction, which usually requires chronic daily drug use, tolerance to the mood elevating or euphoriant effects of the drug frequently occurs (1). Also, after tolerance and addiction have been established, withdrawal occurs if drug use is

Table 1   Mood Effects of Drugs of Abuse

	Status of user		
Drug	Drug naive	In withdrawal	Physiological addict
Alcohol	Euphoria Disinhibition	Anxiety/depression	Relief of anxiety
Cocaine	Euphoria Excitement	Depression	Relief of depression
Heroin	Euphoria	Anxiety/depression	Relief of anxiety

discontinued for a few hours or days. The drug is then used to prevent the unpleasant effects of withdrawal, and often, larger doses are required to obtain a euphoriant effect. Eventually the drug is used to avoid negative mood states, with little or no euphoria experienced. This process is summarized in Table 1.

The addict is in a state of continuous mild withdrawal, even with continuing drug use. Therefore, the mood effects of chronic habitual drug abuse can be conceptualized as resulting in the development of an organic mood disorder.

II.   ORGANIC MOOD DISORDER

''The essential feature of this syndrome is a prominent and persistent depressed mood, resembling a major depressive episode, that is due to a specific organic factor. If the mood is depressed, these features may include fearfulness, anxiety, irritability, brooding, excessive somatic concerns, panic attacks, suspiciousness, and a tearful, sad appearance'' (2). Although this syndrome is conventionally associated with endocrinopathies, use of antihypertensive medication, stroke, viral illness, and other medical provocations, a case can be made for depression associated with chronic substance use. Regarding the secondary depression of alcoholism and drug addiction as an organic mood syndrome or disorder may help the clinician formulate and implement a more effective diagnostic and treatment plan.

Similar to the clinical overlap between primary depressive and anxiety disorders is the overlap between organic mood disorder and organic anxiety disorder. The Diagnostic and Statistical Manual (third edition) (DSM-III-R) lists the use of psychoactive substances as a common etiologic factor in organic anxiety disorder. Typically, anxiety can be caused by stimulant intoxication and by sedative withdrawal. Furthermore, as noted by DSM-III-R, organic mood syndrome may coexist with organic anxiety syndrome, and both diagnoses may be given concurrently.

Habitual chronic substance abuse inevitably alters lifestyle patterns. Substance abusers neglect proper nutrition and, because of intoxication and poor judgment, are at increased risk for infectious disease and trauma. Nutritional deficiencies, infectious disease, and head injury can each cause an organic mood disorder individually. Therefore, finding a persistent depressed mood in a person with a history of substance abuse presents the clinician with a complex and often difficult challenge.

A. Organic Mood Disorder and Substance Abuse

Mood disorders in substance abusers represent a broad area that encompasses many systems. The substance abuser is at increased risk from the direct toxic effects of the substances, from dangerous situations resulting from poor judgment, and from deterioration of general health related to lifestyle. The definition of an organic mood disorder states that the mood symptoms need to be prominent and persistent. The symptoms should be related etiologically to a specific organic factor evident from history, physical examination, or laboratory evidence. A number of studies show that 10%–30% of patients admitted to an inpatient alcohol treatment program are depressed (3). Most of these depressive symptoms resolve after a period of abstinence, although some may persist. It should be emphasized that up to 60% of patients admitted to inpatient substance abuse programs have a diagnosable personality disorder, often with antisocial or borderline features (4). This helps account for the often high-risk behavior associated with substance abuse. Also, depression is a common comorbidity in these personality disorders.

In general psychiatric populations, at least 12% of the patients have an undiagnosed organic condition related to their psychiatric diagnosis

(5). It is therefore necessary to maintain a high index of suspicion for organic causes of mood disorder in substance abusers. All patients should have a thorough medical history, good physical examination, and routine laboratory studies. These should include a complete blood count, liver enzymes, serological test for syphilis, urinalysis, and possibly a test for human immunodeficiency virus (HIV). Depending on the results, and on the history and physical examination, these studies may be expanded. Organic affective disorder can have the same symptoms of depression and mania that will appear in other cases, with the same increased risk for suicide. It should also be noted that patients with a family history of mood disorder appear to be more susceptible to organically induced episodes. Possibly, this is a predisposition that can be precipitated by a variety of factors, both psychological and physical.

The question of why a significant proportion of substance abusers present with a depressive syndrome that resolves with time, and without specific treatment, remains to be answered. Some studies have shown that 15%–40% of alcoholics presenting to inpatient substance abuse programs were clinically depressed at the time of admission, and that approximately three-fourths of these depressions clear with 2 to 3 weeks of sobriety (3). Other studies have shown that 70% of opiate addicts in active treatment are depressed, and that 30% of patients in a maintenance treatment program met criteria for depression (6). After detoxification, if depression persists, the question of whether there are other organic causes of this mood disorder in addition to the substance abused must be answered. Again, the study showing that approximately 12% of all psychiatric patients have an organic cause or contribution to their illness that often goes undiagnosed should be kept in mind (5). In this chapter, we will examine particular factors for which substance abusers may be at risk. However, first we will look closely at substances of abuse, both as toxins and on their effect on neuronal systems involved in depression.

1. Neurochemical Effects of Alcohol

Alcohol is the most widely abused substance in the United States; much research has been done on it. Many reports have documented the changes in neurotransmitter release or metabolism after administration of ethanol to animals and humans. Some of these changes are probably secondary to an induced disruption of ion channels that control the excitability of the neurons. It is important to remember that, although each neurotransmitter system is separate, there are many interactions that influence other neuronal systems. Thus, the differentiation between primary and secondary effects of alcohol on neurotransmitter systems becomes difficult to evaluate.

There has been a great deal of interest in the serotonergic systems of the brain and the effects of alcohol on *serotonin* (5-HT) in both acute and chronic states. A correlation between serotonin and impulsive, violent, and suicidal behavior has been postulated (7), and it is especially important to evaluate this in the substance abusing population. Recent data indicate that acute administration of high doses of ethanol is accompanied by a rise in 5HIAA, the 5-HT metabolite in the brain. There is a reduction or no change in levels of 5-HT at the same time, so it can be concluded that acute ingestion of ethanol increases release or turnover of 5-HT. During withdrawal, this seems to be reversed, at least in animal models, because 5-HT turnover is decreased (8). These serotonergic processes in the brain to chronic ethanol appear to be reversible, since 5-HT turnover is normalized several days after cessation of ethanol (9). Available laboratory data on serotonergic activity in the brains of human alcoholics show some similarity to observations with animals bred to prefer alcohol. However, it is confused by individual variation, which may point out genetic patterns of brain function and behavior.

Synthesis, release, and metabolism of *norepinephrine* in the presence of acute or chronic alcohol ingestion has been the subject of several studies. Low-to-moderate doses of ethanol increase the rate of catecholamine synthesis in laboratory animals; but the levels of norepinephrine are not affected. In human studies, Borg (10) showed that increases of methoxyhydroxyphenylethylglycol in cerebral spinal fluid were found after injection of ethanol in healthy male volunteers. A possible interpretation of these findings might be that, initially, low doses of ethanol increase the rate of norepinephrine synthesis and turnover. As levels of alcohol rise, it appears the norepinephrine neuron activity and norepinephrine turnover begin to be suppressed. Chronic ethanol exposure reportedly increases norepinephrine turnover (11). The metabolites of norepinephrine are elevated throughout the period of observable withdrawal symptomatology and continue to be elevated even after symptoms of withdrawal have cleared. This seems to indicate that the increased norepinephrine activity after withdrawal is not a reaction to stress, nor is it the primary neurochemical determinant of ethanol withdrawal.

High doses of ethanol given in an acute dose cause an increase in activity of tyrosine hydroxylase, which is the rate-limiting step in the production of norepinephrine and *dopamine.* This effect is most marked in the dopamine-rich areas of the brain of mice and rats. The increase in dopamine synthesis is accompanied by a corresponding increase in the metabolites of dopamine (11). It could, therefore, be concluded that the acute ingestion of ethanol stimulates dopamine release from dopamine neurons and the necessary replenishment through increased dopamine synthesis. Tolerance develops with chronic ingestion, and this seems to enhance dopamine turnover. In mice and rats, the tolerance is fully developed after 7 days of daily intake (11). Withdrawal in human alcoholics is accompanied by reduced cerebral spinal levels of dopamine metabolites, which indicates that dopamine turnover is decreased in comparison to individuals not showing withdrawal (12). Thus, decreased dopamine activity may correlate with withdrawal symptoms in humans. Furthermore, dopamine agonists appear to decrease some ethanol withdrawal symptoms in humans (13).

Sleep stages are affected by ethanol and by ethanol withdrawal. Rapid eye movement (REM) sleep and dreaming are suppressed by ethanol (14). Continued ethanol intake will cause some tolerance to this effect, but upon cessation, an abrupt rebound occurs with marked increase in REM sleep. This may be the only sleep stage obtained just before the onset of delirium tremens. The hallucinations of delirium tremens may represent this type of dream state in waking hours. Although much work remains to be done on sleep and alcohol, major sleep disturbances appear to be associated with ethanol withdrawal and its clinical manifestations.

Conventionally, ethanol is thought to exert its intoxicating effect by its action at the g-aminobutyric acid (GABA) receptor, where it facilitates the effects of GABA (15). Patients with alcoholism have low levels of GABA in plasma (16), similar to those seen in patients with primary unipolar major depression (3). Thus, the GABA system provides another dimension of neurochemical commonality between alcoholism and depression.

The kindling theory, developed by Bollinger and Post (17) from their work in mice and rats, may be applied to the hyperexcitement or hyperexcitability of the limbic system after repeated withdrawal from ethanol. This could account for the seizures often seen during withdrawal. Perhaps the brain can be sensitized to the depressant effects of alcohol as well, such that response to psychological stress causes a response that is similar to the depressive effects of the alcohol (18). This could be another factor involved in the observed depression in alcoholics after withdrawal from alcohol.

2. Neurochemical Effects of Heroin

When considering opiate addiction, it should be remembered that opiates are basically central nervous system depressants, although they are often thought to elevate mood because the acutely cause a sense of well-being or euphoria. Therefore, although use of opiates might be considered to be a response to depression or ''self-medication,'' opiate use in and of itself eventually causes long-standing depressive mood changes. Whereas the acute administration of heroin produces euphoria, chronic administration results in depression, hostility, irritability, and agitation. It may be that addicts who use heroin have a shorter course of depression than patients receiving methadone (6). Methadone is a much longer-acting opiate and as such, may cause a more profound impact on the endogenous opiate systems of the brain. This could explain a greater prevalence of major depression in methadone patients compared with heroin addicts. Whether this is a prolonged withdrawal state or continued disruption of the brain mechanisms by the longer-acting opiate in the so-called chronic abstinence syndromes is unknown. Even after acute withdrawal symptoms have abated, depression persists for 2 weeks or longer, along with a number of the symptoms of depression, such as difficulty sleeping, irritability, decreased energy, and anhedonia. The insomnia is easily documented and can persist for months. There is a dose-dependent relationship, with greater symptomatology shown in patients who have been on higher doses vs lower doses of methadone. In the 1970s, research began on the naturally occurring opiate receptors in the brain, which then led to the discovery of the opiate peptides, including the endorphins and enkephalins (19). There are specific neurons in the brain that utilize the endorphins and enkephalins as neuro-modulators and neurotransmitters. These are thought to involve regulation of pain perception and responses to stress and mood that are altered in patients with an opiate addiction. Indeed, the endorphins and enkephalins have been found to show abnormal neuroendocrine responses in patients with depression.

3.   Neurochemical Effects of Cocaine

Recently, interest in this topic has grown. The drug apparently increases the release of dopamine and norepinephrine into the synapse and blocks the reuptake of the substances. With chronic use, this leads to a deficiency of dopamine presynaptically, a result that has been shown in animal studies. The findings of elevated dopamine metabolites in plasma of recently detoxified cocaine addicts support this. The lowered level of dopamine and norepinephrine in the brain is probably one of the contributing factors in high depression rating scale scores among withdrawing cocaine addicts (20). This would account for the immediate depressive ''crash'' in the acute phase of cocaine withdrawal and the period of time needed for the system to adjust (21). The noradrenergic deficit presumed to occur with chronic cocaine abuse forms the neurochemical rationale for treatment of these patients with noradrenergic tricyclic antidepressants such as desipramine (22).

B.   Nutritional Deficiency

Next we will discuss the role of nutritional deficiencies commonly seen in substance abusers. Nutritional deficiencies can occur in populations that appear to maintain a high standard of nutrition. Clearly, individuals abusing substances are more likely to have inadequate or unbalanced nutritional intake, which may predispose them to vitamin deficiencies. The specter of Wernicke's encephalopathy, for instance, looms large in the minds of those involved in the care of alcoholics, a group that presents, a special challenge. Alcoholics often have poor nutritional intake in addition to increased demands on their vitamin reserves for the metabolism of large amounts of alcohol and poor absorption of nutrients from the bowel. However, other substance abusers have similar risks. In organic affective disorders, the B vitamins are most likely to be deficient, particularly thiamine, nicotinic acid, and pyridoxine. Vitamin B_{12} and folic acid have also been shown to have an effect on psychiatric illness. The B vitamins are necessary for carbohydrate glucose metabolism in the brain, and therefore are essential to adequate nerve impulse transmission. The problem of vitamin B deficiencies may be more common than might be suspected in a general psychiatric inpatient population. One study showed that among consecutive patients admitted to an inpatient unit, 30% were thiamine deficient, 27% were riboflavin deficient, and 9% were pyridoxine deficient (8). Although patients often had multiple vitamin deficiencies, at least half showed some evidence of vitamin B deficiency, even though they were from a relatively affluent community.

Thiamine deficiency is probably the vitamin deficiency most associated with alcohol abuse. It is usually considered in terms of its neurological complications, such as Wernicke's encephalopathy, which results from an acute thiamine deficiency and is diagnosed by a triad of findings—global confusion, ophthalmoplegia, and ataxia. However, various studies have demonstrated that in the presence of thiamine deficiency, there will be a progressive change in symptoms that can mimic an affective disorder. A study done in the early 1940s showed that participants maintained on a diet adequate in nutrients except for thiamine had initial development of generalized weakness and depression, decreased appetite, and difficulty sleeping (23). Some also had difficulty concentrating and poor memory, whereas others reported euphoria and paresthesias. Diets that were less deficient over a longer period resulted in emotional lability with irritability and depression in addition to somatic complaints. When adequate thiamine was added back into the diet, these symptoms disappeared. Another study in the late 1950s demonstrated the psychological effects of thiamine deficiency, including weakness, anorexia, irritability, and depression (24). Minnesota Multiphasic Personality Inventory testing on these thiamine-deficient subjects showed elevated hysteria, hypochondriasis, and depression scales. Manual skills and reaction time were impaired, but general intelligence was unaffected.

Vitamin deficiencies are very difficult to study in isolation. It is thought that a deficiency of *nicotinic acid* is primary in pellagra, which would be an extreme example of this problem. The classic triad of manifestations of pellagra are gastrointestinal disorders, skin lesions, and psychiatric disturbances. The psychiatric features of pellagra, which are assumed to be primarily caused by a nicotinic acid deficiency, consist of a general deterioration in mental as well as physical health, with a feeling of incapacity for thinking or acting upon thoughts. Difficulty with appetite and sleep, irritability, and lability are also early manifestations of nicotinic acid deficiency. Depression can be a major problem, with suicide a possibility. More severe nicotinic acid deficiencies can lead to a psychosis with paranoia and to hallucinations, as well as to disorientation and confusion. Administration of nicotonic acid will reverse these symptoms within a matter of days (25).

There have been various studies and observations relating to *pyridoxine deficiency* in humans. Probably the most acute reaction is the seizures that infants who are not receiving adequate pyridoxine may have. Adults given pyridoxine antagonists have demonstrated decreased energy, lability, irritability, and some confusion. With the more sophisticated laboratory analyses currently available, a deficiency of pyridoxine has been shown to contribute to mood disorders, especially depression (26). In fact, on inpatient psychiatric units, deficiencies of pyridoxine, and perhaps riboflavin, have been shown to be greater in patients with mood disorders than in those with other mental disorders. Pyridoxine deficiency is also linked to depression in women taking oral contraceptives.

A deficiency in *riboflavin* produces increased tearing and sensitivity to light, glossitis, and angular stomatitis. The deficiency has also been linked with changes in the Minnesota Multiphasic Personality Inventory, primarily increases in depression, hysteria, and hyperchondriasis (27). Patients on experimental riboflavin-deficient diets showed decreased energy, increases in the number of minor somatic complaints, and hypersensitivity. With the additives available in the modern diet, riboflavin deficiency would be a slowly developing condition.

The classic example of B_{12} *deficiency* is pernicious anemia, which may be accompanied by various neurological complications. However, the earliest symptoms of the anemia are depression and decreased energy, which progresses to increased lethargy or hypersomnia, with apathy when the anemia is more severe. Other psychiatric disorders have been attributed to this deficiency besides mood disorders (28). These include schizophrenia, paranoia, and delirium with dementia, all of which have responded dramatically to B_{12} replacement. Because neuronal loss may be associated with B_{12} deficiencies, it is important to recognize and treat this as early as possible. Although B_{12} requirements are very small and a long period of time would be required to become vitamin deficient from poor diet alone, B_{12} deficits can be accentuated by low folic acid or serum folate (29). Whereas B_{12} deficiencies are more marked in patients who have had gastric lesions, such as alcoholics with chronic gastritis, they should not be overlooked in any of the substance abusing populations with inadequate diets.

The last vitamin deficiency discussed will be *folic acid,* which has been reviewed recently in the literature, and which can result in an anemia of the megaloblastic type, as does B_{12} deficiency. Barbiturates and alcohol, as well as other drugs, can depress serum folate levels. One study showed that of 100 patients with severe depressive illness, 25% were found to have serum folate below 2.5 ng/mL per milliliter (30). Another outpatient study found that patients with lower serum folate had more affective morbidity that those with normal folate levels (31,32).

These data point out that inadequate diet, substance abuse, and dietary deficiencies are strongly associated with organic affective disorders. Considering the high risk of vitamin deficiency in a substance abusing population, these patients should be treated with vitamin supplementation on a routine basis. This may be done by giving a daily multivitamin and a folate supplement orally. Thiamine should be replaced with intramuscular injections of 100 mg daily for at least the first 3 days and then with daily oral supplements. This strategy can prevent complications arising acutely from vitamin deficiency. It will also help correct current deficiencies and perhaps speed recovery from organic mood disorders in the substance abusing population.

C. Infectious Disease

Two major infections need to be considered in the assessment of mood disorders in substance abusing patients. The first is *neurosyphilis,* which has long been considered the ''great imitator'' in medicine. Syphilis has been in decline for many years, but it has seen a recent resurgence in its primary form coinciding with the epidemic of crack cocaine use. The second is HIV infection, which has become a major problem for the general population and for the substance abusing population in particular. These infectious diseases will be briefly discussed, but their treatment is probably best referred to specialists in infectious diseases.

The treatment of syphilis was radically improved with the introduction of penicillin. However, its widespread use for many other infections may have led to early inadequate treatment of syphilis and, consequently, a later incomplete and atypical appearance of neurosyphilis (33). Neurosyphilis can be divided into three different types: general paresis, tabes dorsalis, and meningovascular syphilis. Walton (34) suggested that of any 12 patients with neurosyphilis, five are likely to have general paresis, four, meningovascular syphilis, and three, tabes dorsalis. Of these, general paresis is the most important to us.

General paresis probably first appeared in France after the Napoleonic wars and was spread along trade routes. The cause of general paresis was unknown for many years, but interestingly enough, one of the causes that was postulated was alcohol excess. This was before the discovery of the *Treponema pallidum* bacterium in the early 20th century (35). General paresis in and of itself is thought of as a dementing process, but the early changes may be in personality or mood before any cognitive changes are evident. Several forms of general paresis may be seen. There is a grandiose form, a simple dementive form, a depressive form, a taboparetic form, and other forms with a primarily psychotic presentation. The most common, according to Dewhurst (36), is the depressive form, found in approximately 27% of patients. These appear with all the classic symptoms of depression, including occasional suicidal ideation. There may be a delusional component to this disorder. Its primary distinguishing feature is shallowness of affect with corresponding shallowness of mood detectable on mental status examination. The grandiose form of general paresis is probably becoming less common, although it is still found in cultures other than westernized societies. The clinical presentation is quite striking, with patients being very boastful and expansive, bragging of wealth, sexual powers, or the belief that they are famous people from the past. Often, the patient will make no complaint when hospitalized. However, again, a shallowness of affect and a naive quality to the expansive mood resulting from the ongoing dementia process may be detected. Diagnosis can be made by serological tests and by the assessment of cognitive function and physical examination.

The classic signs of neurosyphilis include the Argyll Robertson pupil, which consists of a small irregular pupil with atrophy of the iris. It reacts to convergence but not to light. A coarse, irregular tremor may be seen in more than 60% of patients on first presentation, usually involving the face and the hands. Approximately 80% have a dysarthria, probably secondary to the tremor of the lips and tongue. The speech is described as slurred, jerky, and irregular. The tendon reflex abnormalities that are seen include exaggerated knee and ankle jerks and clonus in the lower limbs (37). There is some controversy about the treatment of neurosyphilis, but a total of at least 600 million units of penicillin should probably be given. There does not seem to be a need to administer the penicillin directly into the spinal fluid.

Infection with HIV is increasing throughout the world. Those experiencing the greatest increase in new infection are the intravenous (I.V.) substance abusers and their partners. The risk is compounded when the I.V. drug abuser also smokes crack cocaine. There is a documented increase in high-risk sexual behavior in crack cocaine smokers, which is particularly problematic in women who have a large number of sexual partners (38). Probably all substance abusers are at increased risk for HIV, either because they lack judgment while intoxicated with the substance, or because of activities such as prostitution that may be related to obtaining the substance of abuse.

Studies have shown that large percentages of patients with acquired immune deficiency syndrome (AIDS) had evidence of brain involvement (39). It may be that HIV infection is this generation's new ''great imitator'' because of the many ways in which it manifests. Neuropsychiatric presentations of HIV can be depression, mania, or dementia (40,21). The same caveats that applied in neurosyphilis probably apply in HIV infection as well. Because the underlying process in dementing, there is often a shallowness of mood and affect. This is an ongoing process, and the symptoms will change over time. It is likely that cognitive impairment caused by HIV infection will be found if a diligent search is made (41,42). With the immune suppression of the illness, there are other possible infections that can affect the central nervous system. Options for treatment at this time are limited; however, it appears that azidothymidine (AZT) in doses of 600–1200 mg per day will cross the blood–brain barrier and may provide some improvement in the neuropsychiatric position (42). Again, the treatment of HIV is best managed by an infectious disease specialist.

D. Head Injury

The substance abusing population is at high risk for *head injuries* whether from driving while under the influence of substances, falling while intoxicated, or poor judgment while under the influence of substances. Major depression resulting from a closed head injury has about the same incidence as depression after stroke, which is reported in about 27% of cases (43). The psychological morbidity varies widely depending especially on the area injured and the severity of the trauma. Some of the hypotheses for the psychiatric changes include direct interruption of the catecholamine and cholinergic mechanisms, pituitary involvement with resultant neuroendocrine disturbance, and disrupted arousal effect in the mesencephalon. Injury of the left anterior cortex has the highest association with depression, followed by parietal, occipital, and right hemispheric lesions. Other studies suggest that on long-term follow-up, among patients with a penetrating brain injury, those with right-sided injury were more likely to suffer depression. One study of severe head injuries found that only five of 22 patients were free of psychiatric complications from their head injuries, with depressive disorders the most common psychiatric syndrome. There have been reports of good response to serotonin uptake inhibitors (44), although theoretically, patients should respond to tricyclics if they can tolerate the side effects. Involvement of the hypothalamus appears to predispose patients to manic illness. These should be treated appropriately with mood stabilizer drugs. Manic disorders should be differentiated from disinhibition such as occurs in frontal lobe syndromes. However, it is essential to refer to the physical examination for any neurological complications.

III. TREATMENT GUIDELINES

First, the patient must abstain from intoxicating substances. If a physiological addiction has developed, appropriate medication should be used to make the patient safe and comfortable during acute withdrawal. For alcohol addiction, this would usually involve a benzodiazepine. For opiate addiction, clonidine should be sufficient. Acute cocaine withdrawal does not require medication in most instances. As soon as the acute withdrawal period is over, usually in 3–5 days, the medication used to treat the withdrawal should be rapidly tapered and discontinued. This period is particularly difficult for all concerned as the patient may be experiencing many, sometimes drastic, changes—biochemical, physiological, psychological, and social.

Often the physician will be asked to continue an anxiolytic medication after treatment of acute withdrawal. Such requests are best denied inasmuch as good clinical practice requires a drug-free observation period of at least 2 weeks before an accurate diagnosis can be made. It is worth noting that in research protocols, a drug washout of 2 weeks before diagnosis or symptom rating is standard. It is also worth noting that several clinical studies have found that the dysphoria associated with alcoholism will largely to abate with 2 to 4 weeks of sobriety and supportive care (3). Most depressed, recently detoxified substance abusers will not need antidepressant medication because, in most cases, the depression will be transient and remit spontaneously. The patient, who may be quite distressed and insisting on medication, should be told that a period of observation and assessment with no use of any psychoactive substances, whether prescription or otherwise, is needed for an accurate diagnosis.

During this evaluation phase, a careful physical and laboratory examination should be performed, including a complete blood count, blood chemistry, urinalysis, serological tests for syphilis and HIV, and computed tomography (CT) or magnetic resonance imaging (MRI) scan of the head, as indicated by history and clinical presentation. Patients should be instructed in the principles of nutrition, including consultation with a registered dietitian if indicated. During this period of careful medical and psychological evaluation, the physician should also review patients' medications. Those who suffer from substance abuse or dependence are likely to have medical problems such as gastritis, peptic ulcer disease, and hypertension. Some medications used for these general medical conditions can cause a depressive syndrome that may further complicate the picture. Cimetidine, beta-blockers such as propranolol, and methyldopa are particularly associated with depression. Every attempt should be made to manage the medical condition with newer and less toxic agents in these cases.

What if the patient meets criteria for major depressive disorder after 2–4 weeks of abstinence? Then the diagnosis of depression should be made, and the patient should be treated. There is very little by way of scientific data from randomized clinical trials to help in selecting treatment for this secondary depression in abstinent substance abusers. However, clinical experience suggests that standard antidepressant treatments are usually effective in these patients. For mild-to-moderate levels of depression in which the patient is still able to maintain function and receive treatment on an outpatient basis, a trial of either cognitive/ behavioral psychotherapy or antidepressant medications should be undertaken, with close follow-up, usually at weekly intervals. There should be a reassessment of how well depressive symptoms have responded to treatment after 6 weeks (45). The decision whether to treat with medication or psychotherapy should be discussed with the patient. Many alcoholics and drug addicts will prefer to avoid ''pills,'' and this decision should be respected with the proviso that the patient accepts treatment with medication if there is no clear clinical response after a reasonable trial of psychotherapy.

The increasing acceptance of the disease model of addictive behavior and of the biochemical model of depression and other mental illnesses has made the use of medication in treating depression in the addict more acceptable. However, the clinician should be aware that many traditional substance abuse treatment modalities, including some Alcoholics Anonymous and Narcotics Anonymous groups, discourage use of any psychotropic medications in substance abusers. The patient should be assured by the physician that antidepressant medications are not ''addictive,'' are not controlled substances, and will be used for a limited period of time only.

Probably the serotonin uptake inhibitor antidepressants have some therapeutic advantages in the treatment of depressed alcoholics because they are nonsedating, generally well tolerated, and may decrease relapse to alcoholism (46). The tricyclic antidepressants increase the permeability of the blood–brain barrier to alcohol (47). If an alcoholic patient relapses to drinking while taking a tricyclic medication, he may be at increased risk for paradoxical intoxication and blackouts, even with relatively small amounts of alcohol.

If there is no clinical response to the first antidepressant medication used, the patient should be changed to a different class of medication. For example, if the patient fails a trial of serotonin uptake inhibitor, desipramine or bupropion represent logical alternatives. If there is no response to two different classes of antidepressants at full therapeutic doses verified by therapeutic blood monitoring for a 6 to 12 week trial, the diagnosis should be reconsidered, with consultation if necessary. If the diagnosis of major depression is confirmed and abstinence from drugs of abuse is documented, augmentation therapy with lithium should be considered. If this fails, electroconvulsive therapy may be needed. If there is a response to antidepressant medications with remission of symptoms, treatment should be continued at full dose for 6 months after clinical response. The medication should then be tapered, with follow-up for an additional 6 months to observe for possible recurrence of depression.

IV. SUMMARY

This has been a brief overview of a large area of organic mood disorders that occur in a substance abusing population; however, it is by no means exhaustive. The direct toxic effects of substances have been considered, as well as the complications of poor health habits and risk-taking behavior that the substance abuser exhibits. The importance of a good history, thorough physical examination, and routine laboratory work cannot be overemphasized. Supportive care, follow-up with good nutrition, and augmentation with proper vitamin supplements should be considered routine. The combination of length of abstinence, good physical and laboratory examinations, adequate nutritional support, and coordinated efforts among appropriate medical specialists will assure the best possible outcome in this population.

REFERENCES

1. S. Perry, and J. Markowitz, *Textbook of Psychiatry* (J. Talbott, R. Hales, and S. Yudofskysled, eds.), American Psychiatric Press, Washington, D.C., 1988, pp. 279–312.
2. American Psychiatric Association (APA), *Diagnostic and Statistical Manual of Mental Disorders* (3rd ed. rev.), Washington, D.C., 1987.
3. F. Petty, *Gen. Hosp. Psychiatry 14:*258–264 (1992).
4. E. Nace and P. Isbell, *Clinical Textbook of Addictive Disorders* (R. Frances and S. Miller, eds.), Guilford Press, New York, 1991, pp. 43–68.
5. D. A. W. Johnson, *Practitioner 200:*688–691 (1968).
6. I. Extein, C. A. Dackis, M. S. Gold, and A. L. C. Pottasit, *Medical Mimics of Psychiatric Disorder,* American Psychiatric Press, Inc., Washington, D.C., 1986, p. 131.
7. A. Roy, M. Virkkunen, and M. Linnoila, *Int. J. Neurosci. 41:*261–264 (1988).
8. D. Nutt, and P. Glue, *Br. J. Addict. 81:*327–338 (1986).
9. J. C. Ballenger, F. K. Goodwin, L. F. Major, and G. L. Brown, *Arch. Gen. Psychiatry 36:*224–227 (1979).
10. S. Borg, H. Kvande, D. Mossberg, P. Valverius, and G. Sedvall, *Pharmacol. Biochem. Behav. 18:*375–378 (1983).
11. P. L. Hoffman and B. Tabakoff, *Alcohol and the Brain: Chronic Effects* (R. E. Tarter, D. H. Van Thiel, and K. L. Edwards, eds.), Plenum Press, New York, 1985, p. 19.
12. L. F. Major, J. C. Ballenger, F. K. Goodwin, and G. L. Brown, *Biol. Psychiatry 12:*635–642 (1977).
13. S. Borg, and T. Weinnholdt, *Acta Psychiatr. Scand. 65:*101–111 (1982).
14. N. Imatoh, Y. Nakazawa, H. Ohshima, M. Ishibashi, T. Yokoyama, *Drug Alcohol Depend. 18:*77–85 (1986).
15. M. K. Ticku, *Ann. Med. 22:*241–246 (1990).
16. F. Petty, J. Steinberg, G. L. Kramer, M. Fulton, and F. G. Moeller, *J. Affect. Disord. 29:*53–56 (1993).
17. R. M. Post, D.R. Rubinow, and J. C. Ballenger, *Br. J. Psychiatry 149:*191–201 (1986).
18. R. M. Post, *Am. J. Psychiatry 149:*999–1010 (1992).
19. S. H. Snyder, *Am. J. Psychiatry 135:*645–652 (1978).
20. C. Dackis, and M. Gold, *Neurosci. Biobehav. Rev. 19:*469–477 (1985).

21. L. R. Dickson, and J. D. Ranseen, *Hosp. Community Psychiatry 41*:290–300 (1990).
22. F. Gawin, and E. Ellimword, *Annu. Rev. Med. 40*:149–161 (1989).
23. R. D. Williams, H. L. Mason, M. H. Power, and R. M. Wilder, *Arch. Intern. Med. 71*:38–53 (1943).
24. J. Brozek, and W. O. Custer, *Am. J. Clin. Nutr. 5*:109–120 (1957).
25. T. D. Spies, C. D. Aring, J. Gilperin, and W. B. Bean, *Am. J. Med. Sci. 196*:461–475 (1938).
26. M. W. P. Carney, A. Raindran, M. G. Rinsler, and D. G. Williams, *Br. J. Psychiatry 141*:271–272 (1982).
27. R. T. Sterner and W. R. Price, *Am. J. Clin. Nutr. 26*:150–160 (1973).
28. D. K. Zucker, R. L. Livingston, R. Nakra, and P. J. Clayton, *Biol. Psychiatry 16*:197–205 (1981).
29. R. Shulman, *Br. J. Psychiatry 113*:252–256 (1967).
30. M. W. P. Carney, *Br. Med. J. 4*:512–516 (1967).
31. R. D. Williams, H. L. Mason, R. M. Wilder, and B. F. Smith, *Arch. Intern. Med. 66*:785–799 (1940).
32. A. Coppen, and M. T. Ahou-Saleh, *Br. J. Psychiatry 141*:87–89 (1982).
33. H. Hooshmand, and B. W. Browley, *JAMA 219*:726–729 (1972).
34. J. N. Walton, *Brain's Disease of the Nervous System*, Oxford University Press, London, 1977, p. 136.
35. E. H. Hare, *J. Med. Sci. 105*:594–626 (1959).
36. K. Dewhurst, *Br. J. Psychiatry 145*:612–619 (1969).
37. W. A. Lishman, *Organic Psychiatry: The Psychological Consequences of Cerebral Disorder*, Blackwell Scientific Publications, Oxford 1987, p. 287.
38. R. Booth, J. Watters, D. Chitwood, *Am. J. Public Health 83*:1144–1148 (1993).
39. S. Perry, and P. Jacobsen, *Hosp. Community Psychiatry 37*:135–142 (1986).
40. M. Faulstich, *Am. J. Psychiatry 144*:551–556 (1987).
41. S. Perry, *Am. J. Psychiatry 147*:696–710 (1990).
42. F. L. Wilkie, C. Eisdorfer, R. Morgan, D. A. Lowenstein, and J. Szapocznik, *Arch. Neurol 47*:433–440 (1990).
43. J. Fedoroff, S. E. Starkstein, A. W. Forrester, F. H. Geisler, R. E. Jorge, S. V. Arndt, R. G. Robinson, *Am. J. Psychiatry 149*:918–923 (1992).
44. R. Bessette, and L. Peterson, *Psychosomatics 33*:224–226 (1992).
45. Depression Guideline Panel, *Depression in Primary Care: Volume 2. Treatment of Major Depression. Clinical Practice Guidelines, Number*

5, Rockville, MD, U.S. Department of Health and Human Services, Public Health Service, Agency for Health Care Policy and Research, AHCPR Publication No. 93-0551, April 1993.

46. J. M. Murphy, M. B. Waller, G. J. Gotte, W. J. McBride, L. Lumeng, and T. K. Li, *Alcohol 5:*283–286 (1988).

47. D. W. Goodwin, *J. Psychiatr. Treat. Eval. 5:*445–450 (1983).

8

Treatment for Seasonal Affective Disorder (SAD)

Raymond W. Lam
University of British Columbia and Vancouver Hospital and Health Sciences Centre, Vancouver, British Columbia, Canada

I. INTRODUCTION

A decade ago, a group of researchers at the National Institute of Mental Health identified a series of patients who had recurrent depressive episodes during the winter. Since Rosenthal and colleagues (1) published these initial cases of seasonal affective disorder (SAD) in the *Archives of General Psychiatry,* there has been a tide of research into SAD. This disorder is now widely accepted in the psychiatric community as a subtype of recurrent depression, and it has been included in the Diagnostic and Statistical Manual (DSM)-III-R and the DSM-IV, where it is categorized as a "course specifier" for recurrent mood disorders.

More recently, there has been increasing interest in the connection between seasonality and substance abuse. There are several case reports of seasonal patterns in alcoholism and cocaine abuse, both often associated with seasonal depressions (2–4). One obvious explanation is that these may simply be spurious associations. Inasmuch as both SAD and substance abuse are common disorders, it would not be surprising to find patients suffering from both disorders concurrently. Patients who increase their drinking or substance abuse to "self-medicate" against their winter depression may then appear to have a seasonal pattern of abuse. However, other studies have found that patients with SAD more often have a family history of alcoholism in first-degree relatives than patients with nonseasonal depression (5). This suggests a genetic relationship of the two disorders that goes against a simple coincidence phenomenon. Some studies have shown that pineal melatonin levels show seasonal variability in alcoholic subjects, and some of the neuropsychiatric effects of cocaine may also be mediated through the pineal body (3,6). These findings offer the intriguing suggestion that substance abuse may be associated with seasonal biological factors. Some investigators have suggested that eating disorders belong to an addictive disease spectrum. Seasonal patterns of bulimia nervosa have been identified, and up to 30% of bulimic patients experience winter worsening of their mood and eating symptoms (7,8). The seasonality of addictive disorders and their relationships to SAD therefore appear to be a fruitful area for further research.

Much of the research interest in SAD has been spurred by its novel treatment by bright light exposure, or light therapy. In this chapter, I will review current knowledge about the therapeutic effects of light in SAD, the current clinical protocol for light therapy used in our clinic, and other treatments for SAD.

II. LIGHT THERAPY FOR SAD

Using light to treat depression is not a new concept. Dr. J. H. Kellogg, for example, wrote a book in 1913 entitled *Light Therapeutics* in which he recommended "arc lights and buttermilk" for the treatment of melancholia (9). Unfortunately, Kellogg's light therapeutics (unlike his corn flakes) did not survive the era. It was not until 1980, when Al Lewy and colleagues reported that light had biological effects on human melatonin secretion (10), that light exposure was studied again in treatment of mood disorders. As early as 1981, Kripke reported the first controlled trials of bright light exposure for depression, although he was studying nonseasonal depression (11). The first case studies of light therapy for SAD were reported in 1982 (12).

Since the first reports of light therapy, various parameters of thera-peutic light have been studied, including wavelength, intensity, time of day, and duration of exposure. Most light therapy studies have used light boxes composed of a bank of fluorescent tubes. Intensity of light exposure has traditionally been measured by lux, a unit of illumination. Controlled studies using light boxes have shown that intensities of 500 lux or less are not effective in treating SAD, compared with light of 2500 lux or more (13). Although 500 lux is considered "dim light" relative to 2500 lux, it is equivalent to bright office lighting and, therefore, is a reasonable control condition. In comparison, indoor social lighting rarely exceeds 100 lux. The light outdoors on a cloudy day, even during winter, is usually in the 4000 lux range, whereas sunny days can reach intensities of 50,000 to 100,000 lux or more.

Although early studies used so-called "full-spectrum" fluorescent tubes, many studies have subsequently shown that other light sources are equally effective, including cool-white fluorescent tubes and incan-descent bulbs (14,15). Wavelength studies have shown that green light seems to be slightly more effective than narrow-wavelength red or blue light, although white light seems to be the most effective (16–18).

There also appears to be a relationship between intensity and duration of exposure. Earlier studies using 2500 lux light boxes required 2 hours of daily exposure for optimal response (19). However, the newer 10,000 lux light boxes require only 30 minutes of light exposure to achieve similar response rates (20,21). The timing of light therapy continues to be a controversial subject. Based on circadian rhythm hypotheses, morning light exposure should preferentially correct the postulated phase-delayed rhythms in SAD. Several studies have found superiority in morning light (20, 22–24), but other studies have not (25,26). Some studies show good response rates even with midday or evening exposure (27,28). A grouped analysis of pre-1990 studies found that morning light had a significantly higher response rate compared with evening light (53% vs 37%) (13).

The original light boxes were large, heavy, and awkward to use. The latest generation of light boxes are small, lightweight, and portable and are now available from a number of commercial sources. Because illumination, as measured by lux, falls with the inverse square of the distance, the newer light boxes achieve a higher lux rating simply by placing the light source much closer to the subject (within 18 inches). The use of a stand that positions the light box above and at an angle to the subject avoids the problem of glare that exists with a direct-facing light source.

A.   A Method for Light Therapy

The following is the light therapy protocol that we use in our clinic. This regimen is based on data from controlled clinical studies, but we recognize that other centers may use slightly different methods.

We currently recommend using light boxes that provide 10,000 lux of illumination. We instruct patients to start with 30 minutes of light exposure upon awakening at about 7:00 AM. Patients should also try to sleep and wake at regular times. The patients sit under the light box, which is on a desk stand. The antidepressant effect is mediated through the eyes (29), so patients must be awake with their eyes open, but they can read or eat breakfast and do not need to stare at the lights (Figure 1). If there is little response after 2 weeks, we suggest increasing the duration of exposure to 60 minutes, or switching to evening light exposure (e.g., from 7:00 PM to 8:00 PM). If evening exposure is used, patients should not use the lights too near bedtime, because sleep can be disrupted by late evening bright light exposure. Patients typically begin to notice antidepressant effects after 3 to 5 days of exposure, and the clinical response is usually apparent within 2 weeks. However, patients will also relapse within the same time period if the light exposure is stopped. Thus, most patients with SAD need to continue daily light therapy during the winter months when they are usually depressed, and to stop light therapy in the spring. Occasionally, patients will also use the light box during dark or cloudy days in the spring and summer.

B.   Efficacy of Light Therapy

The response rate for light therapy in SAD varies from 50%–90% depending on the criteria used to define clinical response. In our clinic, we have treated SAD outpatients using 10,000 lux light therapy in a standardized, open protocol. Patients were assessed by experienced

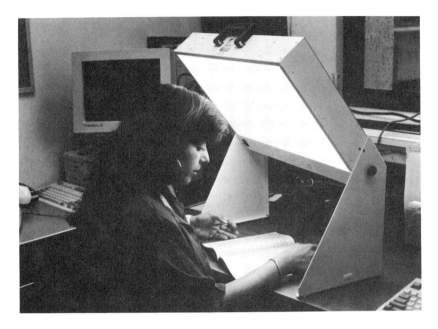

Figure 1   A 10,000 lux light box used for the treatment of seasonal affective disorder.

psychiatrists using unstructured clinical interviews. Diagnoses are assigned using DSM-III-R criteria, and all diagnoses are routinely verified with a chart review by a research psychiatrist. All patients met DSM-III-R criteria for recurrent major depressive episodes with a seasonal pattern (equivalent to SAD). Patients taking antidepressant medications were eligible if they had taken the medications for at least 6 weeks and were still symptomatic. No dose changes were allowed during the light therapy trial. After a baseline week, patients used a light box at home daily for 2 weeks. The light therapy consisted of a 10,000 lux, cool-white fluorescent light box (SunBox Company, Bethesda, MD) with 30 minutes of exposure upon awakening at 7:00 AM. Patients were assessed weekly with the Structured Interview Guide for the Hamilton Depression Rating Scale, Seasonal Affective Disorder version (SIGH-SAD) (30). The SIGH-SAD incorporates the traditional 21-item Hamilton Depression Rating Scale (HDRS) (31) and an 8-item atypical addendum that rates the atypical depressive symptoms frequently seen in patients with SAD, including hypersomnia, hyperphagia, carbohydrate craving, and weight gain. Compliance was checked weekly by inspection of sleep/mood logs.

We studied 68 patients with SAD during two winters, from 1991 to 1993. Table 1 shows the demographic variables for the patients. The majority of patients had unipolar depression as previously reported by us and others (32,33). All members of our sample group met DSM-III-R criteria for recurrent major depression and may have been more seriously affected than samples reported at other centers. Certainly, a high proportion of our patients had previous psychiatric contact (75%) and past treatment with antidepressant medications (69%).

Table 2 shows the results of the course of light therapy. There are statistically significant reductions in all the depression scores after 2 weeks of light therapy. The mean percentage improvement in the 29-item SIGH-SAD score was 57% (±25% SD), with a range of improvement of 4%–98%.

Although the results show clear statistical significance, the clinical significance of response is also important to consider. If clinical response is defined as greater than 50% reduction in the SIGH-SAD scores, then 62% of these patients were responders to light therapy.

Table 1 Demographic Information for SAD Patients (N = 68)

Diagnosis	
Unipolar Depression	90%
Bipolar, Type I	3%
Bipolar, Type II	7%
Gender	
Female	71%
Male	29%
Age at Assessment	37.2 ± 10.3 years
Previous Depressive Episodes	10.7 ± 7.9
Past Psychiatric History	
Psychiatric Contact	75%
Medication Use	69%
Hospitalization	16%

Table 2   Results from 2-Week Trial of Light Therapy (N = 68 subjects)

Measure	Baseline	Post-Treatment[1]
HDRS[2], 17-item	17.1 ± 3.4	6.6 ± 4.6
HDRS, 21-item	19.4 ± 3.9	7.6 ± 5.2
Atypical Addendum[3]	13.1 ± 4.9	6.1 ± 4.0
SIGH-SAD[4]	32.5 ± 6.1	13.7 ± 7.9
Beck[5]	26.0 ± 8.4	10.8 ± 8.4

[1]All results significant at $p < 0.0005$; paired t-tests, df = 67.
[2]Hamilton Depression Rating Scale.
[3]Atypical Symptom Addendum, 8-item.
[4]Structured Interview Guide for the Hamilton Depression Rating Scale, Seasonal Affective Disorder version, 29-item.
[5]Beck Depression Inventory.

Using Terman's more stringent criteria for clinical remission (greater than 50% reduction in the 21-item HDRS *and* a posttreatment HDRS score of less than 8), then 63% of patients were remitters. Side effects were minimal; approximately 15% of patients had mild headaches, and 6% had mild nausea. None had to discontinue light therapy because of troublesome side effects.

These results need to be interpreted with caution because of the open design of the study, and controlled studies may have lower response rates (34). However, the response seen in this large clinical sample suggests that the 10,000 lux protocol is clinically beneficial for a majority of patients with SAD.

Terman et al. (13) published a grouped analysis of 29 studies using light therapy protocols, usually of 2500 lux for 2 hours. They concluded that the strictly defined remission rate from light therapy was 53% for bright light, but only 11% for dim light. However, most studies to date have only investigated short-term use of light therapy during a period of 1 to 2 weeks. Predictors of response to light therapy have also been studied by several groups (35–37). The atypical depressive symptoms of hyperphagia, increased weight, and hypersomnia appear to be significantly associated with light therapy response across studies.

Although there is consensus that light therapy is effective, the magnitude of the placebo effect of light therapy remains a scientific issue

(38). As others have remarked, light is an obvious treatment that makes sense to patient with SAD, and the light itself cannot be disguised, so a true "double-blind" study cannot be done. Previous studies have attempted to control for nonspecific or expectation effects by using dim light or by using deception. A recent study attempted a novel approach by using a negative ion generator (which, unknown to subjects, was inactivated) as a control condition. Eastman and colleagues did not find a significant difference between the ion generator and a bright light condition (7000 lux for 1 hour at 7:00 AM for 2 weeks) (39). However, whereas the negative ion generator condition had a response rate of 25% (similar to that of dim light controls in light box studies), the bright light condition had a response rate of only 29%, much lower than any previous light therapy studies. The reason for the low bright light response is unclear. Therefore, the extent of placebo or nonspecific effects in the use of light therapy for SAD remain unresolved.

C. Light Therapy Devices

A number of other types of light devices are now marketed for light therapy. These can be divided into categories of light visors, other head-mounted devices (e.g., light glasses), dawn simulators, and miscellaneous devices. Of these, only the light visor (which uses a rechargeable, battery-operated incandescent light source) and the dawn simulator have been studied in controlled clinical trials. Light visors appear to reduce SAD symptoms to a similar degree as light boxes, although no direct comparative studies have been done. However, several studies involving the largest sample sizes of light therapy subjects to date have been unable to demonstrate an intensity-response relationship for the light visor (40–42). Therefore, very dim light (e.g., 60 lux) appears to be as effective as dim light (400 to 600 lux) and bright light (3200 to 6000 lux). This may indicate that light visors are more effective because of the proximity of the light source to the eye, that lux is not the relevant measure of the biological or therapeutic effects of light, or that light visors have large placebo effects. Despite this controversy, these three studies do support that light therapy using light visors provides marked relief for about 60% of patients with SAD.

The dawn simulator device slowly increases ambient lighting in a bedroom in the early morning while patients are sleeping to simulate a summer dawn (43). Several preliminary reports suggest that the dawn simulator may also be effective in treating SAD, despite a final illumination of only 250 lux (44–46).

Other devices have not undergone scientific study, and there is little regulation of light therapy devices in most countries. Because the essential parameters for delivery of light in light therapy are still unknown, a conservative approach to treatment is indicated. Light devices that have not been studied in controlled clinical trials should be used with caution. Similarly, we do not recommend that patients build their own light boxes because of the electrical hazards involved and the inaccurate dosing of light.

D. Side Effects of Light Therapy

Few side effects are experienced by most patients with properly conducted light therapy. About 20% of patients complain of headaches, eyestrain, or feeling "buzzed" during the light exposure (47). These side effects are usually mild or respond to reducing the duration of exposure. Bipolar I patients may experience abrupt switches to hypomania, so light therapy should be used with caution in these patients, especially if they are not treated with a mood stabilizing medication such as lithium. As a precautionary note, we have seen one patient who may have "overdosed" on light. He had previously had unipolar winter depressions but used his 10,000 lux light box for 3 to 4 hours a day and became psychotically manic, requiring hospitalization. Although this may have been the result of a spontaneous switch into mania in a previously unrecognized bipolar patient, the use of light may not be as innocuous as we would like to believe.

There is some controversy among researchers in SAD about the need for routine ophthalmological evaluation in patients before beginning light therapy (48,49). Potential hazards of light exposure include ultraviolet exposure and bright light toxicity. Although fluorescent lighting emits only small amounts of ultraviolet rays, the constant and recurrent exposure of light therapy can lead to lifetime exposures that are in the toxic range. Because the ultraviolet spectrum (< 400 nm) is not required for the antidepressant effect (50), light therapy devices should include a screen that blocks all wavelengths below 400 nm. Bright light exposure of 10,000 lux intensity is not generally considered to have toxic effects on the retina. However, bright light may potentiate the effects of photosensitizing medications, including lithium and the neuroleptics, or may exacerbate a preexisting retinal condition such as macular degeneration (51). Some reassuring data include a recent follow-up study of light therapy in patients with SAD that found no clinical or electrophysiological evidence of eye damage after 5 years (52). Mandatory ophthalmological evaluation prior to light therapy is probably not necessary, but ophthalmological assessment and regular follow-up should be done in: 1) patients with preexisting eye disease (e.g., glaucoma, retinal disease, cataract surgery); 2) patients with systemic diseases that can involve the retina (e.g., diabetes); 3) patients taking highly photosensitizing medications (e.g., lithium, antipsychotic drugs, chloroquine); and 4) elderly patients.

E. Mechanism of Light Therapy

When SAD was first described, there was much hope that an etiology would soon be discovered because of the apparent link between a plausible animal model of seasonality (photoperiodism) and a rational treatment (bright light). Unfortunately, research to date has highlighted that SAD is likely a heterogenous condition, and no clear pathophysiology for SAD and the therapeutic effects of light has emerged. Major theories include circadian rhythm abnormalities, reduced retinal light sensitivity, and dopaminergic or serotonergic dysfunction.

Animals are obviously much more seasonal in their behavior than humans. Seasonal patterns of animal behaviors, such as reproductive activity, are mediated through daily changes in the light/dark cycle (photoperiodism). These animal models of photoperiodism led to suggestions that circadian rhythm disturbances may result in the seasonal mood, sleep, and appetite symptoms seen in SAD. Since the light/dark cycle, or photoperiod, is the strongest zeitgeber (synchronizer) of circadian rhythms in mammals, the therapeutic effect of bright light may be mediated through a corrective effect on human circadian rhythms (53). In this hypothesis, the timing of light therapy is critical, because animal and human data have shown that the direction and magnitude of circadian phase shifts are dependent upon the time of exposure. Indeed, some groups have shown phase-delayed rhythms of core body temperature and melatonin secretion in patients with SAD that are corrected by appropriately timed light exposure (22,24,54). However, other studies have not been able to replicate these results (25,26,55). Some studies have shown that patients with SAD have reduced light sensitivity in winter at the level of the retina, as measured by electroretinography and electrooculography, compared with controls (56–58). This may explain why these patients require a larger ''dose'' of light in the winter to synchronize their circadian rhythms. There are conflicting results, however, on whether these retinal changes are corrected by light therapy (58,59). Still other studies using different retinal electrophysiological measures found no differences between SAD and controls (60).

Despite some of these conflicting studies of SAD, it is now clear that bright light exposure does have predictable effects on human biological rhythms (61). Thus, there is active research on the use of bright light in chronobiological disorders such as phase-delayed sleep disorder, jet lag, and shift-work disorders.

Other neurobiological studies have found evidence for dysregulation of dopamine and serotonin in SAD. Low basal serum prolactin levels and reduced eye blinks may suggest hypodopaminergic function in SAD, which is not altered by light therapy (62,63). Serotonin is of interest in SAD because it is a neurotransmitter that has a robust seasonal pattern of secretion in humans, with lowest levels in the winter/spring, and highest levels in summer/autumn (64). The finding that behavioral and hormonal responses to a serotonergic challenge such as m-chlorophenylpiperazine are abnormal in SAD has been replicated by the same group (65). These abnormal responses are corrected after light therapy. There is at least preliminary evidence that light may have a direct effect on serotonin receptors (66).

In summary, there is promising research on the mechanisms of light therapy, especially in regard to the circadian and serotonergic effects of light. At this point, however, the antidepressant mechanism of light therapy remains to be proven conclusively.

III.   OTHER TREATMENTS FOR SAD

Treatment with light has received the most research interest in SAD, and it may be somewhat surprising that more traditional treatments for depression, such as medications, have not been well studied. In part, practical factors make it more difficult to study the effects of antidepressants in SAD. Most antidepressant studies require at least 6 weeks of treatment, with a week or two of medication washout/baseline monitoring. The window to enter subjects for a 6-week treatment study of SAD is narrow; recruitment cannot extend past mid-February to ensure that natural spring remission by the beginning of April is not a confounding factor. Thus, the recruitment window is a narrow 4 months from mid-October to mid-February.

Only small case series and open studies have been reported for medication treatment of SAD. These studies suggest that SAD responds to antidepressant medications such as tranylcypromine (67) and bupropion (68), and to serotonergic medications such as d-fenfluramine (69) and l-tryptophan (70). A recent study found that fluoxetine was as effective as light therapy in treating depressed patients with SAD, but that study did not include a true placebo control (71). Two large placebo-controlled, double-blind studies of selective serotonin reuptake inhibitors (fluoxetine and sertraline) have been recently completed in Canada and Europe. Although results are not yet available, they will provide important information about antidepressants in SAD. Another important clinical question that remains unanswered is whether some SAD patients do better on a combination of light therapy and an antidepressant compared with either one alone.

Research in SAD has thus far been focused on biological etiologies and treatments. As yet, there has been no reported research on psychological therapies for SAD, despite the fact that psychological treatments such as cognitive-behavioral therapy have demonstrated effectiveness in treating depression of unspecified seasonality.

IV.   SUMMARY

Within the past decade, SAD has become widely accepted as a subtype of recurrent depressive disorders, and seasonality is becoming recognized as clinically important in other disorders such as bulimia nervosa. The relationship of seasonality and SAD to substance abuse is another intriguing question that will need further exploration. Light therapy is a safe, effective, and practical treatment for SAD. The role of antidepressant medications is only beginning to be studied in SAD, and there are as yet no studies of psychological treatments for winter depression. Further research is required to tease out the pathophysiology of SAD and seasonality, the mechanism of light therapy, and the optimal treatment of this common depressive subtype.

REFERENCES

1. N. E. Rosenthal, D. A. Sack, J. C. Gillin, A. J. Lewy, F. K. Goodwin, Y. Davenport, P. S. Mueller, D. A. Newsome, and T. A. Wehr, *Arch. Gen. Psychiatry 41:*72–80 (1984).
2. S. L. Satel, and F. H. Gawin, *Am. J. Psychiatry 146:*534–535 (1989).
3. R. Sandyk, and J. D. Kanofsky, *Int. J. Neuroscience 63:*195–201 (1992).
4. R. E. McGrath, and M. Yahia, *J. Clin. Psychiatry 54:*260–262 (1993).
5. J. M. Allen, R. W. Lam, R. A. Remick, and A. D. Sadovnick, *Am. J. Psychiatry 150:*443–448 (1993).
6. A. K. Jain, S. Kelwala, J. Campbell, B. Powell, S. Yerasi, and S. Khoury, "Seasonal Change of Melatonin Rhythm in Alcoholics," New Research Program and Abstracts, 143rd Annual Meeting of the American Psychiatric Association, Washington D.C., 1990, p. 259.
7. R. W. Lam, L. Solyom, and A. Tompkins, *Compr. Psychiatry 32:*552–558 (1991).
8. A. Blouin, J. Blouin, P. Aubin, J. Carter, C. Goldstein, H. Boyer, and E. Perez, *Am. J. Psychiatry 149:*73–81 (1992).
9. D. F. Kripke, D. J. Mullaney, M. R. Klauber, S. C. Risch, and J. C. Gillin, *Biol. Psychiatry 31:*119–134 (1992).
10. A. J. Lewy, T. A. Wehr, F. K. Goodwin, D. A. Newsome, and S. P. Markey, *Science 210:*1267–1269 (1980).
11. D. F. Kripke, *Biological Psychiatry* (C. Perris, G. Struwe, and B. Jansson eds.), Elsevier, Amsterdam, 1981, p. 1248.
12. A. J. Lewy, H. A. Kern, N. E. Rosenthal, et al., *Am. J. Psychiatry 139:*1496–1498 (1982).
13. M. Terman, J. S. Terman, F. M. Quitkin, P. J. McGrath, J. W. Stewart, and B. Rafferty, *Neuropsychopharmacology 2:*1–22 (1989).

14. B. I. Yerevanian, J. L. Anderson, J. L. Grota, and M. Bray, *Psychiatry Res. 18:*355–364 (1986).

15. R. J. Bielski, J. Mayor, and J. Rice, *Psychiatry Res. 43:*167–175 (1992).

16. G. C. Brainard, D. Sherry, R. G. Skwerer, M. Waxler, K. Kelly, and N. E. Rosenthal, *J. Affect. Disord. 20:*209–216 (1990).

17. D. A. Oren, G. C. Brainard, S. H. Johnston, J. R. Joseph-Vanderpool, E. Sorek, and N. E. Rosenthal, *Am. J. Psychiatry 148:*509–511 (1991).

18. K. T. Stewart, J. R. Gaddy, B. Byrne, S. Miller, and G. C. Brainard, *Psychiatry Res. 38:*261–270 (1991).

19. A. Wirz-Justice, A. C. Schmid, P. Graw, K. Krauchi, P. Kielholz, W. Poldinger, H. U. Fisch, and C. Buddeberg, *Experientia 43:*574–576 (1987).

20. J. S. Terman, M. Terman, D. Schlager, B. Rafferty, M. Rosofsky, M. J. Link, P. F. Gallin, and F. M. Quitkin, *Psychopharmacol. Bull. 26:*3–11 (1990).

21. A. Magnusson, and H. Kristbjarnarson, *J. Affect. Disord. 21:*141–147 (1991).

22. A. J. Lewy, R. L. Sack, L. S. Miller, and T. M. Hoban, *Science 235:*352–354 (1987).

23. D. H. Avery, A. Khan, S. R. Dager, G. B. Cox, and D. L. Dunner, *Acta Psychiatr. Scand. 82:*335–338 (1990).

24. R. L. Sack, A. J. Lewy, D. M. White, C. M. Singer, M. J. Fireman, and R. Vandiver, *Arch. Gen. Psychiatry 47:*343–351 (1990).

25. T. A. Wehr, F. M. Jacobsen, D. A. Sack, J. Arendt, L. Tamarkin, and N. E. Rosenthal, *Arch. Gen. Psychiatry 43:*870–875 (1986).

26. A. Wirz-Justice, P. Graw, K. Krauchi, B. Gisin, A. Jochum, J. Arendt, H.-U. Fisch, C. Buddeberg, and W. Poldinger, *Arch. Gen. Psychiatry 50:*929–937 (1993).

27. S. P. James, T. A. Wehr, D. A. Sack, et al., *Br. J. Psychiatry 147:*424–428 (1985).

28. F. M. Jacobsen, T. A. Wehr, R. A. Skwerer, D. A. Sack, and N. E. Rosenthal, *Am. J. Psychiatry 144:*1301–1305 (1987).

29. T. A. Wehr, R. G. Skwerer, F. M. Jacobsen, D. A. Sack, and N. E. Rosenthal, *Am. J. Psychiatry 144:*753–757 (1987).

30. J. B. W. Williams, M. J. Link, N. E. Rosenthal, and M. Terman, *Structured Interview Guide for the Hamilton Depression Rating Scale, Seasonal Affective Disorders Version (SIGH-SAD),* New York State Psychiatric Institute, New York, 1988.

31. M. Hamilton, *Br. J. Soc. Clin. Psychol. 6:*278–296 (1967).

32. R. W. Lam, A. Buchanan, and R. A. Remick, *Ann. Clin. Psychiatry 1*:241–245 (1989).
33. D. M. White, A. J. Lewy, R. L. Sack, M. L. Blood, and D. L. Wesche, *Compr. Psychiatry 31*:196–204 (1990).
34. C. I. Eastman, *Psychopharmacol. Bull. 26*:495–504 (1990).
35. D. A. Oren, F. M. Jacobsen, T. A. Wehr, C. L. Cameron, and N. E. Rosenthal, *Compr. Psychiatry 33*:111–114 (1992).
36. K. Krauchi, A. Wirz-Justice, and P. Graw, *Psychiatry Res. 46*:107–117 (1993).
37. R. W. Lam, *Acta Psychiatr. Scand. 89*:97–101 (1994).
38. M. C. Blehar, and A. J. Lewy, *Psychopharmacol. Bull. 26*:465–494 (1990).
39. C. I. Eastman, H. W. Lahmeyer, L. G. Watell, G. D. Good, and M. A. Young, *J. Affect. Disord. 26*:211–221 (1992).
40. R. T. Joffe, D. E. Moul, R. W. Lam, A. J. Levitt, M. H. Teicher, B. Lebegue, D. A. Oren, A. Buchanan, C. A. Glod, M. G. Murray, et al., *Psychiatry Res 46*:29–39 (1993).
41. M. H. Teicher, C. A. Glod, D. A. Oren, C. Luetke, P. Schwartz, C. Brown, and N. E. Rosenthal, ''The Phototherapy Light Visor: There is More to It Than Meets the Eye,'' Abstracts of the 4th Annual Meeting of the Society for Light Treatment and Biological Rhythms, Wilsonville, OR, 1992, p. 20.
42. N. E. Rosenthal, D. E. Moul, C. J. Hellekson, D. A. Oren, A. Frank, G. C. Brainard, M. G. Murray, and T. A. Wehr, *Neuropsychopharmacology 8*:151–160 (1993).
43. M. Terman, D. Schlager, S. Fairhurst, and B. Perlman, *Biol. Psychiatry 25*:966–970 (1989).
44. D. Avery, M. A. Bolte, and M. Millet, *Acta Psychiatr. Scand. 85*:430–434 (1992).
45. D. H. Avery, M. A. Bolte, S. Cohen, and M. S. Millet, *J. Clin. Psychiatry 53*:359–363 (1992).
46. D. H. Avery, M. A. Bolte, S. R. Dager, L. G. Wilson, M. Weyer, G. B. Cox, and D. L. Dunner, *Am. J. Psychiatry 150*:113–117 (1993).
47. A. J. Levitt, R. T. Joffe, D. E. Moul, R. W. Lam, M. H. Teicher, B. Lebegue, M. G. Murray, D. A. Oren, P. Schwartz, A. Buchanan, et al., *Am. J. Psychiatry 150*:650–652 (1993).
48. C. E. Reme, and M. Terman, *Am. J. Psychiatry 149*:1762–1763 (1992).
49. M. Waxler, R. H. James, G. C. Brainard, D. E. Moul, D. A. Oren, and N. E. Rosenthal, *Am. J. Psychiatry 149*:1610–1611 (1992).

50. R. W. Lam, A. Buchanan, J. A. Mador, M. R. Corral, and R. A. Remick, *J. Affect. Disord. 24:*237–243 (1992).

51. M. Terman, C. E. Reme, B. Rafferty, P. F. Gallin, and J. S. Terman, *Photochem. Photobiol. 51:*781–792 (1990).

52. C. P. Gorman, P. H. Wyse, S. Demjen, L. H. Caldwell, M. Y. Chorney, and N. P. Samek, ''Ophthalmological Profile of 71 SAD Patients: A Significant Correlation Between Myopia and SAD,'' Abstracts of the 5th Annual Meeting of the Society of Light Treatment and Biological Rhythms, Wilsonville, OR, 1993, p. 8.

53. A. J. Lewy, R. L. Sack, C. M. Singer, D. M. White, and T. M. Hoban, *J. Biol. Rhythms 3:*121–134 (1988).

54. K. Dahl, D. H. Avery, A. J. Lewy, M. V. Savage, G. L. Brengelmann, L. H. Larsen, M. V. Vitiello, and P. N. Prinz, *Acta Psychiatr. Scand. 88:*60–66 (1993).

55. C. I. Eastman, L. C. Gallo, H. W. Lahmeyer, and L. F. Fogg, ''Searching for Clues to SAD in the Circadian Rhythm of Temperature,'' Abstracts of the 5th Annual Meeting of the Society for Light Treatment and Biological Rhythms, Wilsonville, OR, 1993, p. 6.

56. R. W. Lam, C. W. Beattie, A. Buchanan, R. A. Remick, and A. P. Zis, *Am. J. Psychiatry 148:*1526–1529 (1991).

57. R. W. Lam, C. W. Beattie, A. Buchanan and J. A. Mador, *Psychiatry Res. 43:*55–63 (1992).

58. N. Ozaki, N. E. Rosenthal, D. E. Moul, P. J. Schwartz, and D. A. Oren, *Psychiatry Res. 49:*99–107 (1993).

59. R. W. Lam, C. W. Beattie, J. A. Mador, M. R. Corral, A. Buchanan, and A. P. Zis, ''The Effects of Light Therapy on Retinal Electrophysiologic Tests in Winter Depression,'' Abstracts of the 5th Annual Meeting of the Society of Light Treatment and Biological Rhythms, Wilsonville, OR, 1993, p. 10.

60. D. A. Oren, D. E. Moul, P. J. Schwartz, J. R. Alexander, E. M. Yamada, and N. E. Rosenthal, *Depression 1:*29–37 (1993).

61. C. A. Czeisler, J. S. Allan, S. H. Strogatz, J. M. Ronda, R. Sanchez, C. D. Rios, W. O. Freitag, G. S. Richardson, and R. E. Kronauer, *Science 233:*667–671 (1986).

62. R. A. Depue, W. G. Iacono, R. Muir, and P. Arbisi, *Am. J. Psychiatry 145:*1457–1459 (1988).

63. R. A. Depue, P. Arbisi, S. Krauss, W. G. Iacono, A. Leon, R. Muir, and J. Allen, *Arch. Gen. Psychiatry 47:*356–364 (1990).

64. V. Lacoste, and A. Wirz-Justice, *Seasonal Affective Disorders and Photo-*

therapy, (N. E. Rosenthal, and M. C. Blehar, eds.) Guilford Press, New York, 1989, p. 167.

65. J. R. Joseph-Vanderpool, F. M. Jacobsen, D. L. Murphy, J. W. Hill, and N. E. Rosenthal, *Biol. Psychiatry 33:*496-504 (1993).

66. R. Mason, *Seasonal Affective Disorder,* (C. Thompson, and T. Silverstone, eds.), CNS (Clinical Neuroscience), London, 1989, p. 243.

67. S. C. Dilsaver, and R. S. Jaeckle, *J. Clin. Psychiatry 51:*326–329 (1990).

68. S. C. Dilsaver, A. B. Qamar, and V. J. Del Medico, *J. Clin. Psychiatry 53:*252–255 (1992).

69. D. O'Rourke, J. J. Wurtman, R. J. Wurtman, R. Chebli, and R. Gleason, *J. Clin. Psychiatry 50:*343–347 (1989).

70. R. E. McGrath, B. Buckwald, and E. V. Resnick, J. Clin. Psychiatry 51:162–163 (1990).

71. S. Ruhrmann, S. Kasper, B. Hawellek, B. Martinez, G. Hoflich, T. Nickelsen, and H. J. Moller, *Biol. Psychiatry 33:*83A (1993).

9

Cognitive Therapy of Depression During Addiction Recovery

Norman Cotterell
University of Pennsylvania, Philadelphia, Pennsylvania

I. INTRODUCTION

This chapter will focus on the cognitive therapy of depression in addiction recovery as a way to conceptualize a patient's problem areas and to plan therapeutic technique and strategy. Beck and his colleagues first designed cognitive therapy for the treatment of depression (1). Later work extended it to the treatment of anxiety disorders, somatoform disorders, eating disorders, substance abuse, and personality disorders (2,3). As a treatment model, it offers structure, ease of conceptualization, and empirical validation. It offers a theoretical model that bridges the gap between theory and practice. This chapter will first examine how depression can play a role in addiction recovery.

II. DEPRESSION IN ADDICTION RECOVERY

The course of recovery is not smooth. Two-thirds of patients relapse within 3 months of treatment (4). Individuals in recovery contend with anxiety, anger, conflict, and family problems. They face joblessness, homelessness, crime, and violence. Any of these could lead the way to lapse and relapse.

Prochaska and his colleagues describe five stages of recovery (5). Depression can be a factor in any of these stages.

Precontemplative stage: The users do not admit that using is the problem. They may believe that using is the solution to their problems.

Contemplative stage: They consider using to be a problem, but cannot stop on their own.

Preparation: They intend to stop using but do not know how to start.

Action: They decrease their activity and start to change their beliefs.

Maintenance: They work to remain consistent in living a drug/alcohol–free life.

In any of these stages, individuals may hold negative beliefs about themselves, their personal world, and their future. In the *precontemplative stage,* individuals may feel powerless to face the problems in their lives. In the *contemplative* and *preparation stages,* they may feel unable to resist drugs or alcohol. In the *action* and *maintenance stages,* they may face the loss of their former lifestyle and friendships. They may feel helpless in sustaining the changes in their lives. In any of these stages, individuals may regard themselves as unloveable, out of control, or inadequate. They may regard others as powerful, controlling, rejecting, inconsiderate, or corrupt, and they may believe that their future is hopeless, destined for poverty, lonely, fruitless, and bleak. They can attribute their dysphoria to themselves, their addiction, or to the problems they hope to solve by getting drunk or high.

III. COGNITIVE MODEL OF DEPRESSION

The cognitive model provides a road map by which a therapist can describe a patient's problem, design strategy, and devise interventions. It presents points at which therapists can focus, intervene, and assess

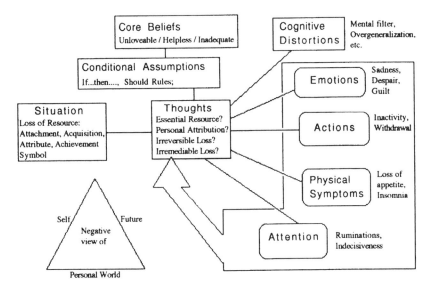

Figure 1 Cognitive model of depression.

progress. The specific model of depression, as outlined below, points to major factors of depression.

Depression is a syndrome thought to have biological, psychological, and social etiology. It exhibits physical and psychological symptoms, such as feeling down, worthless, or guilty, having fewer interests, an inability to enjoy previously pleasurable activities, lack of sleep or sleeping too much, fatigue, lack of energy, agitation, and change in eating patterns, usually a lack of appetite.

Triggers are activating events, circumstances that can be internal (physical sensations, emotions), external (unemployment), or interpersonal (an argument). They prompt feelings and actions that, in turn, can influence other people and circumstances and thereby trigger still more feelings and actions.

Thoughts reflect how individuals interpret such triggers given their biases, beliefs, and assumptions. *Automatic thoughts* are the actual and subtly perceived contents of these thoughts. The therapist asks the patient, ''What was going through your mind when you felt angry?''

Beliefs are general principles patients hold about themselves (their internal resources, skills, talents, vulnerabilities), their personal world (its general status, the risks present in it, the people who make it up), and their future (their chances for happiness, competence, loveability, control, and change).

Assumptions are conditional beliefs. Such beliefs allow patients to cope with a changeable world. They define the conditions (if someone rejects me, if I perform poorly on the job . . .) of one's beliefs (. . . I am unlovable, worthless, incompetent).

Emotions are the subjectively experienced expression of mood. The patient feels happy, sad, angry, scared, frustrated, anxious, or guilty. Such moods are the markers of automatic thoughts. By attending to, focusing on, and querying emotions, therapists can uncover key automatic thoughts.

Physical symptoms may accompany changes in mood. Fatigue, exhaustion, loss of appetite, and sleeplessness can coincide with depression. Challenging and threatening circumstances can trigger autonomic nervous arousal. The resultant symptoms are sweating, trembling, heart rate increase, dry mouth, flushing, pallor, dizziness, and faintness. Such sensations can themselves be challenging or threatening circumstances.

Attention refers to miscellaneous cognitive processes: concentration, memory, self-focus, or hypervigilance. This concerns what patients focus on and how they do so.

Cognitive distortions are systematic ways that people adjust information to make it consistent with their core beliefs. Typical distortions as described by Burns (6) are mental filter, all-or-none thinking, magnification/minimization, ''should'' statements, emotional reasoning, fortune telling/mind reading, personalization/blame, disqualifying the positive, overgeneralization, and labeling.

A. Triggers

This section will cover the typical triggers of depressive mood within the context of drug and alcohol addiction. Although the causes of depression remain elusive (7), episodes can arise from a variety of circumstances: internal (changes in health), external (financial difficulties), and interpersonal (fights, conflicts).

Triggers are the immediate antecedents of dysphoria, as well as physical sensations, cravings, and behaviors. They are situations that awaken core beliefs and assumptions. They reflect sensitivities and start self-perpetuating patterns. They are grounded in an individual's environment, based on interactions with others, or formed within one's own body. Depressive triggers often hold a common theme—loss. Circumstances that trigger depressive episodes involve loss perceived to be permanent, personal (their fault), and pervasive (8). Recovering addicts are no strangers to such loss.

1. Typical Situations That Can Prompt Dysphoria

The kinds of situations that trigger dysphoria typically involve some form of loss. It may be magnified, distorted, or regarded as unchanging, but still such a loss, real or perceived, characterizes depression. A loss of internal attributes, intimate attachments, acquisitions, or signs of achievement and ability can start and maintain a depressive episode.

a. Loss. Individuals recovering from addiction experience loss in many realms. Alcohol, drugs, and addictive behaviors increase the patients' perceptions of their abilities, power, pleasure, and attractiveness. Abstinence can initially mean a loss of those friendships, attachments, and activities that filled their life with meaning. They may lose the friends with whom they got high or the contacts from whom they scored. They may miss the family members who introduced them to drugs and the sexual partners they introduced to drugs. They also lose the attributes and abilities associated with drug use: acceptance by others, sexual power, euphoria on demand, freedom from anxiety, being cool, supreme confidence, excitement, risk, and intrigue. Finally, they lose some of the values that sustained their addiction: immediate short-term gratification over long-term success, sex over intimacy, following the crowd, and love of danger. They may find such values both familiar and seductive. Without anything to substitute for them, patients can lose their grounding—and the base values that gave them identity.

Situations that can remind patients of loss include:

1. They visit an old neighborhood.
2. They see an old friend.
3. They are reminded of past pleasures.
4. They are invited to a party.
5. They are slow on the job.
6. They are bored or inactive.
7. They experience cravings for the addiction.

Any of these circumstances could trigger the negative evaluations of self, personal world, and future that characterize depression.

B.   Cognitions

Cognition refers to the process, as well as the products of thoughts. It refers to what people think about, the interpretations they make, and the way they think. In the cognitive therapy of depression, cognitions are key targets of change. They are the internal experience (words, pictures) of people as they feel and act. They form the bulk of many an intervention. Therapist and patient work together to focus upon, record, examine, classify, respond to, and change them.

As detailed in the literature (9), depressed individuals are likely to make negative interpretations of their daily circumstances. Beck and colleagues (1) have characterized such interpretations as reflecting a depressive triad.

1. *Negative view of self.* Depressed individuals would tend to view themselves as more helpless, incapable, or unlovable than they really are. They perpetuate a negative self-esteem in the way they estimate their own worth, and they continually fall short in their own eyes.
2. *Negative view of their own personal world.* Depressed individuals are prone to viewing their external and interpersonal environment in the negative extreme. They see it as more unloving, rejecting, imposing, or threatening than it really is. To some extent, such individuals influence their environment. Actions

born out of a self-perception of unlovability may prompt rejection. Rejection only confirms that one is unlovable.

3. *Negative view of the future.* Depressed individuals are more likely to see the future as hopeless, grim, and unchanging. Such hopelessness is a key factor in suicide (10,11).

1. Typical Cognitions During Recovery

Recovery can mean loss—of a lifestyle, friendships, or perceived abilities. In addition, people face the potential loss of sobriety in a lapse or relapse. Recovering addicts may regard these lost resources (friendship, ability, sobriety) as essential to their esteem and survival. Depressed individuals, when faced with the loss of an essential resource, may see it as reflecting a personal shortcoming, perhaps their inherent defectiveness. For example, a loss of friendship could mean, ''I'm unlikeable,'' A loss of abilities, ''I can't. Why even try?'' A loss of sobriety, ''I'm just a junkie.''

Secondly, they may expand their own personal shortcoming to pervade their entire personal world. A loss of friendship, ''They have their own lives—no one cares'' A loss of ability, ''Who is gonna help me? I'm alone in this'' A loss of sobriety, ''The deck is stacked against me—what's the point?''

Finally, they may see the loss as permanent and irreversible. A loss of friendship, ''I'm never going to have anyone care for me the way they did'' A loss of ability, ''I'll never be able to work that way again'' A loss of sobriety, ''There's nothing ahead for me—I'm done.''

a. Cognitive Distortions. Cognitive distortions are characteristic ways in which people process information to make it consistent with their depressogenic assumptions. Beck et al. (1) and Burns (6) have classified several of these distortions. *Selective abstraction* involves selecting and focusing on one piece of information to the exclusion of others. *Magnification/minimization* involves stressing the importance of information consistent with one's biases and devaluing information inconsistent with such biases. *Emotional reasoning* involves relying solely on feelings to determine that something is true, to the exclusion of outside evidence. *Fortune telling* is predicting the future based on preconceived biases. *Mind reading* involves divining the motives and

thoughts of others without checking them for validity. *"Should" state-*
ments are unrealistic moral imperatives applied to oneself (often resulting in guilt) or others (often resulting in anger). *Labeling* is attaching
names to oneself or others that are not a true representation of reality.
All-or-none thinking involves seeing circumstances in extremes, not
in degrees.

C. Emotions

Emotions are the subjective markers of cognitions. When a patient
undergoes an upsurge of emotion, the therapist can ask, "What was
going through your mind just then?" The patients learn to use emotions
as signals to attend to any thoughts and images that pass through their
mind. Depression can involve such emotions as sadness, anger, anxiety,
frustration, hopelessness, or guilt.

D. Behaviors

Behaviors are the objective and visible markers of cognition. Key
behaviors, whether procrastination, social avoidance, shouting, or
drinking, can be points where patients attend to their own thoughts,
and where they can plan and consider other means of acting. Typical
behaviors associated with depression are inactivity and withdrawal.
Patients suspend and conserve energy, volition, will, and initiative. They
do this rather than waste such valuable resources on hopeless ventures.

E. Physical Symptoms

Physical sensations can also arise from cognition. Reminders of drug
use can trigger memories of time spent using and the associated physical
sensations of craving, such as tingling, stomach upset, lightheadedness,
etc. Thoughts of threat and harm can contribute to the physical sensations of anxiety: heart rate increase, sweating, trembling, hot flashes,
etc. Depression can be connected to physical symptoms of exhaustion,
loss of appetite, weight loss, or insomnia.

F. Attention

Depression can frame what patients pay attention to and how they
encode, remember, and retrieve information. They may be more likely

to attend selectively and respond extremely to information consistent with their negative biases.

Other depressed patients may have difficulty focusing at all. They experience general cognitive symptoms of depression, such as decreased concentration and drifting attention. When depressed, attention, concentration, and focusing become difficult to maintain. Depressed individuals focus solely on their own perceived debility, their own sense of loss, and their own shortcomings.

IV. TREATMENT MANUAL

A. Therapeutic Relationship

The therapeutic relationship allows the techniques to work. It is an important aspect of therapeutic progress. It allows the patient and therapist to work together to try out a variety of techniques and to experiment with different strategies. It provides a context wherein the beliefs, biases, and assumptions of the patient come into play. The therapist and patient work together to attend to thoughts and emotions triggered in session. The ideal relationship allows this to happen with ease. The therapist builds up rapport, is genuine, generates therapeutic empathy, and thereby forms a trusting relationship. All of this leads to setting a collaborative working relationship.

1. Collaboration

These aspects of the therapeutic alliance create collaboration between therapist and patient. It is a working relationship in which the therapist and patient share responsibility for therapeutic work. They process each agenda item and set goals and priorities. Together, they assess progress and devise homework assignments. Collaboration is key in all these areas.

The therapist and patient work together to face the problem and define key issues. They design goals, treatment plans, and self-help strategies. The therapist notes the commonalities among the patient's thoughts and gradually builds a conceptualization. The therapist explains the rationale behind in-session exercises and homework assignments.

B. Basic Skills

1. *Socratic Questioning*

The process of therapy is the asking of questions. Through questions, therapists explore, investigate, discover, and intervene. As part of collaboration, cognitive therapists ask questions and train patients to ask themselves questions. This helps to maintain an active focus in therapy. The therapist attends to changes in emotion, posture, facial expression, a smile, a tear, or anything that signals change in thought. The therapist asks the patient ''What is going through your mind?'' This question becomes part of the patient's vocabulary. Whenever the patient notices a change in emotion, he or she asks, ''What is going through my mind?''

Therapists also use questions to deepen exploration of issues. Patients seek answers to their problems. Therapists give them an active role in therapy, helping to make them responsible for their own progress. Therapists use questions to teach, present interventions, and ask for feedback.

Typical Questions

What is going through your mind?
How do you see that?
What are the advantages or benefits of doing that? What are the
    disadvantages or costs?
How do you explain that?
What's the meaning of that? What does it mean to you?
What upsets you most about that?

2. Feedback

Therapists must continually determine the patient's understanding of any material presented. They assess the patient's response to the homework assigned, as well as general feelings toward the therapy session, the interventions, and the therapeutic relationship. Therapists cannot assume that the patient's understanding matches their own. Proper questioning can bring out misunderstandings and reservations, as well as insight and revelation.

Typical ways of asking for feedback

What do you hear me saying?
What do you think about what I said?
What do you think about this approach?
How well do you think we work together?
How do you feel about the homework?

C. Structure of the Session

Structuring therapy sessions is essential. Session structure encourages the effective use of time, keeps the session on track, and focuses interventions. The structural elements of a cognitive therapy session are agenda setting, mood/cravings checks, capsule summaries, homework, and constant feedback.

1. Setting the Agenda

The therapist sets the agenda by asking on what particular topics or goals the patient would like to focus. Agenda items can entail mood checks, review of homework assignments, or a check of craving/ urges for drugs and alcohol. They can include assessment of the frequency, duration, and intensity of particular thoughts, emotions, or actions. The patient's agenda items are framed in clear, definable procedures or goals, or in steps that lead to a particular goal. The therapist takes the vague general complaints of a patient and asks questions to crystalize those complaints into clearly defined goals. For example, ''What would you like to see happen? What changes would you like to see in this area?''

> *Therapist:* The first thing we do as part of therapy here is set an agenda. It helps us to keep on track and cover the topics most important to you. For the agenda today, we can review your scores on the depression and anxiety questionnaires you filled out, get some additional background on your problem, and start setting goals. Is there anything else that you would like to put on the agenda?
> *Patient:* Depression, how to stay clean. Just stuff to help me out.

Therapist: Okay, depression. Staying clean. First, with depression. What specifically would you like to accomplish today in regard to your depression?

Patient: I just want to understand what makes me depressed and how to get rid of it.

Therapist: Okay, and about staying clean. What specifically would you like to accomplish today in that area?

Patient: Mainly, how to deal with people from my past. They keep coming by. I don't know what to do. I don't know if I can trust myself.

Therapist: All right, for the agenda today we have (1) going over the questionnaires; (2) setting goals; (3) understanding depression and how to get rid of it; and (4) dealing with people from your past. Is there anything else you'd like to work on today?

Patient: No, that's about it.

Therapist: Okay, where would you like to start?

2. *Mood Checks*

The therapist checks the mood of the patient for signs and symptoms of depression and anxiety. Important questions to ask concern hopelessness and suicidality, general perceptions about themselves, their personal world, their future. Questions can focus on the physical symptoms that accompany emotion and the severity of such symptoms. They can focus on the effort the patient took to cope with them. They can examine whether the patient regarded the symptoms as unbearable or incapacitating. The Beck Depression Inventory (BDI) and Beck Anxiety Inventory (BAI) are helpful for such quick assessments (12,13).

In addition, therapists can devise a quick assessment for other symptoms. They can evaluate the strength and frequency of urges for drugs or alcohol and expected high-risk circumstances. They can examine the frequency, duration, and intensity of worries. In addition, therapists can assess ruminations or obsessions, the frequency of procrastination, and invitations to anger. The only limits to such checks are the specific complaints involved and the combined creativity of therapist and patient.

3. Working Through the Agenda

Each agenda item connects with thoughts, feelings, and actions in the patient's experience. Therapists can help patients examine what is present and develop what is missing. For example, they can help pinpoint internal and external triggers to troublesome thoughts and emotions. They can help patients attend to and recognize their own thoughts and feelings and provide them with a vocabulary with which to label their emotions. Then therapists can ask patients about the behaviors, strategies, physical sensations, words, etc. that follow the thoughts. Finally, they can equip them with methods to examine their own thoughts, beliefs, and behaviors.

a. Situations.   Patients who present thoughts or feelings without context can learn to describe the circumstances, stream of thoughts, and physical sensations that triggered such a response in them. The following shows an example of this.

> *Patient:* I just couldn't function. I felt defeated, hopeless. I didn't want to do anything. I didn't want to—I wanted to see people, to get together with people, but when it didn't happen it was just—I just didn't know what to do. I couldn't do anything. Sometimes I can't do anything.

The therapist can ask: "What was happening right before you started feeling this? What couldn't you do? What brought you down this time?" Questioning can help determine if the triggers were external (interpersonal conflict, poor performance) or internal (stream of thought, remembrances, physical sensations). The therapist helps the patient to connect thoughts, feelings, and behaviors to a particular time and place.

b. Emotions.   Patients who present situations or thoughts devoid of emotions can learn the vocabulary of emotions. Initially, they may harbor notions that make it possible for them to avoid or withhold emotional expression. For example, they might believe that emotional expression shows a lack of control, or that it might prompt rejection by other people.

Patient: When I went to that meeting, I thought the others would judge my behavior, my actions, the general me, what I wear. I said to myself ''Don't say something that sounds foolish. You'll look dopey.''

Open-ended questions can help the patient pinpoint the specific emotions experienced. These emotions may be sadness, fear, anger, or anxiety, or even excitement and joy. For example, a patient is reluctant to state such feelings. The therapist can ask, ''What might happen if you felt this way or expressed this feeling?'' Patients can learn to recognize, report, and detail such emotions. Therapists can help patients test for any catastrophic consequences they fear may result from expressing or experiencing such emotions.

c. Behaviors. Finally, patients can present situations, thoughts, and emotions without presenting any action or behaviors on their part. A patient's actions influence other people and the environment. Likewise, other people and the environment influence the patient. For example, after having a fight with her children, a woman feels angry.

Patient: Where is this coming from? I can't do anything about it. I have no control.

The therapist can simply ask, ''What did you do?'' ''What happened then?'' The therapist must get a sense of what the patient did with her thoughts and emotions. Did she erupt into a verbal assault? Did she withdraw and steam? Each of these strategies follow from beliefs the patient holds of herself, others, her abilities, and her future.

4. Homework

Therapy typically takes place once or twice a week. Often, the most important therapeutic work occurs between sessions. Homework is a way to extend the work of therapy beyond the session. Therapist and patient agree upon, set, revise, and schedule assignments. Typical initial homework involves recording thoughts, scheduling pleasurable or mastery-oriented activities, and testing beliefs. Homework assignments bring the work of therapy home. They give patients the opportunity to put into practice what they learn in session.

The patient's depressive beliefs can sometimes reduce homework compliance. In such cases, the therapist works with the patient to put the ideas (especially of helplessness or hopelessness) to the test. They work together to examine and test the evidence that backs up such beliefs. Even slight modification of such ideas can clear the way for homework compliance.

5. *Capsule Summaries*

Before moving to the next agenda item, the therapist and patient typical review the main points of the current item. The therapist can first detail the situation, thoughts, beliefs, emotions, and behaviors. Then the therapist can review (or have the patient review) the new thoughts, beliefs, and conclusions. In addition, the patient can learn and test new strategies. Preferably, the therapist asks the patient to review these main points and lessons. This enhances the patient's ability to put therapy in to personal language. They understand, remember, and use the new techniques and perspectives covered.

6. *Review*

To summarize, in a typical cognitive therapy session, the therapist:

1. Checks the patient's mood
2. Sets the agenda
3. Works with the patient on the first agenda item and assigns homework
4. Presents a capsule summary
5. Works with the patient on the second agenda item and assigns homework
6. Presents a capsule summary
7. Works with the patient on the third agenda item and assigns homework
8. Offers final summary

Throughout the session, the therapist asks questions to encourage feedback and to explore emotions, automatic thoughts, situations, behaviors, and beliefs.

D. Case Conceptualization

Case conceptualization in cognitive therapy offers a map by which therapy may be guided. The model for depression (negative view of self, personal world, and future) shows the territory at large. The details lie in the case formulation. The therapist pulls together information gathered from interview, diagnosis, family background, and session behavior. From this, the therapist devises hypotheses about what initiates and maintains the patient's difficulties.

1.   Background Data

Core beliefs are forged in childhood. Patients learn about intimacy and responsibility from their parents, about authority from parents and teachers, and about friendship from their peers. These initial experiences help create the notions patients hold about themselves, their place in the world, and their potential. In building a case conceptualization, the therapist examines information that connects with the patient's current difficulties. This information consists of the significant events in the patient's life. Parents, peers, and family members play a role in this. Abuse, neglect, separations, and disasters may act as key events.

Additional details may come out in the initial interview. The therapist pulls together information about: 1) the severity of the patient's depression; 2) whether the patient is psychologically minded; 3) the problems the patient finds most distressing; and 4) the problems most amenable to change. The conceptualization includes all pertinent background information.

2.   Core Beliefs

Core beliefs arise with patients at their most distressed, angry, sad, scared, or upset. They are simple and unconditional: "I am unloveable" "I am weak." They offer clear-cut statements on the patients' view of themselves, their surroundings, their circumstance, and other people. Typical core beliefs include feeling unlovable, unlikeable, lonely, incapable, helpless, and powerless.

3.   Rules and Assumptions

Assumptions are conditional beliefs. They reflect the circumstances, situations, and conditions in which the core beliefs are true or not true. They can be framed as if/then statements, i.e., if I'm broke, I'm powerless; if no one calls me, it must mean I'm unlikeable; if I don't have a man, I'm unlovable.

Patients do not consciously and constantly hold to their core beliefs. These beliefs, although grounded in early experience, are triggered by current circumstances. Loss of a friendship, loss of ability, or loss of a job can unsurface these beliefs. Such circumstances reflect the sensitivities patients have. They are the buttons that get pushed. They are the expectations patients hold about themselves, others, and the world.

"Should" rules are a particular type of assumption that reflect unrealistic or unnecessary expectations about how they, others, and the world should operate. Such statements as, "People should treat me fairly (or else I will do them harm)," or "I should be successful in everything I do (or else I'll regard myself as an abject failure)," are examples of such assumptions.

4. Strategies

These are strategies that patients engage in to deal with the consequences of their beliefs. Such tactics can involve methods that either maintain the dysfunctional beliefs, avoid their consequences, or compensate for the perceived shortcomings. For example, a man may have the core belief, "I am a loser," and the assumption, "To be a winner, I must be admired by all my peers." He may discount any achievements (maintenance), procrastinate from doing work assignments (avoidance), or work compulsively and exaggerate his achievements (overcompensation). Thus, similar core beliefs and assumptions may produce very different strategies. Likewise, very different beliefs and assumptions may produce similar strategies.

E. Techniques

The techniques of cognitive therapy follow from the case conceptualization. The general model of depression suggests that the patient holds a negative view of self, personal world, and future. Therapeutic exercises, activities, experiences, and homework assignments can change such perceptions. For example, common strategies associated with depression are isolation and social withdrawal. Interventions in this area can focus on scheduling activities and increasing social interaction.

Conceptualization helps the therapist determine which techniques are most appropriate to use. Cognitive and behavioral techniques are at the therapist's disposal. For example, depressive beliefs can concern hopelessness, helplessness, and worthlessness. As part of the conceptualization, the therapist examines the flexibility of such beliefs. The more serious and intractable they are, the more likely that therapy will need to start with behavioral techniques to provide the patient with early successes. This experience helps motivate patients to engage in a more thorough examination of their beliefs. The following are some behavioral assignments commonly used in cognitive therapy.

1. Behavioral Techniques

a. Scheduling Activities. Depression saps motivation. Depressed individuals are prone to inertia and may be loathe to act. They may regard all efforts as doomed to failure. Often the first task for a therapist is to increase the level of activity. This, in turn, lifts the patient's sense of efficacy, accomplishment, and enjoyment. The key is to start modestly and work up. Depressed individuals often believe they must feel motivated before they can act. The reverse is actually true. Motivation follows action. Activity schedules are good for assessing and assigning such action.

Initial assignments for depressed individuals often involve the assessment of current activity level and the assignment of activities. Therapists and patients can grade activities according to pleasure or mastery, although any useful qualities can substitute. They use a 1 to 10 pleasure scale to show how enjoyable their daily activities are. They use a 1 to 10 mastery scale to show their level of success at a task, their competence, or just the sense of accomplishment or pride felt in doing it.

The activity schedule lists each hour of the day or night the patient has available. At first the patients list their actual use of time in a given week. Any amount of detail works. The important thing is for them to be aware where their time goes. This sets up a baseline of activity. The patient reports, ''I didn't do anything all week.'' The therapist has a record of time spent. The patient reports, ''I couldn't enjoy a thing.'' The therapist has ratings of a pleasurable walk. The patient reports, ''I accomplished nothing; what little I did was a waste.'' The therapist has ratings of successful presentation.

Recording such activities helps patients be aware of times when they feel competent and experience pleasure. Depressive thinking reduces one's ability to attend to, record, encode, retrieve, and remember positive experiences (9). Having the patient record such experiences helps counteract this.

Activity scheduling can help set future activities. After evaluating a patient's current level of activity, the therapist and patient can then schedule additional activities. Patients may believe they must feel motivated before they can act. The therapist suggests the reverse. Activity scheduling can test this idea that action leads to motivation and then to more action. Patients can check their mood and motivation prior to the scheduled activity. After fifteen minutes or so, they can check it again. They can examine the beliefs triggered and emotions felt. The patient and the therapist can summarize the conclusions and set future activities. Other uses for activity schedules are:

1. For procrastination, patients can schedule tasks and projects. Then they can mark completed tasks with a highlighter.
2. To plan activities, patients can predict the amount of pleasure or mastery they expect. Later, they can rate the actual pleasure or mastery.
3. Patients can plot the time, duration, and intensity of various symptoms, such as headache pain, drug/alcohol cravings, obsessions, and compulsions.
4. Therapist and patient can plan and schedule specific times for homework assignments.

b. Testing New Behaviors. Patients often frame their beliefs as predictions about what they can or cannot do. For example, "I can't speak up for myself," or "I'll fail if I try." The therapist's role is to help the patient put some of these ideas to the test. Patients can test new behaviors to expand their level of activity. They can break old patterns and try out new strategies to replace old ones. For instance, patients may have notions about their own unloveability,and they may avoid starting new relationships or withdraw from existing ones. The therapist, after examining some of the beliefs that maintain such behavior, can prescribe tasks graded from least to most difficult. The least difficult task may be to spend 5 minutes chatting with an intimate, the

	M	T	W	Th	F	S	S
6-7 am							
7-8							
8-9							
9-10							
10-11							
11-12							
12-1 pm							
1-2							
2-3							
3-4							
4-5							
5-6							

	M	T	W	Th	F	S	S
6-7 pm							
7-8							
8-9							
9-10							
10-11							
11-12							
12-1 am							
1-2							
2-3							
3-4							
4-5							
5-6							

Figure 2   Activity schedule.

most difficult task may be to ask an acquaintance out to dinner. The least difficult may be to ask another person's opinion about a television program. A more difficult task may be to reveal one's own feelings to a family member.

Again, the problem behaviors, the obstacles met in changing them, and the thoughts and feelings surrounding them, are all integrated into the cognitive conceptualization. Behavioral goals could involve building new non–drug-oriented relationships, gaining support in twelve-step groups, or applying for work. Other goals could include discovering new non–drug-oriented activities, initiating activities toward greater health, or taking advantage of educational opportunities.

2.   Cognitive Techniques

a.   Eliciting Thoughts.   By definition, cognitive therapists focus intensely on cognition. The therapist focuses on the thoughts, ideas, beliefs, biases, and assumptions that patients hold about themselves, other people, and their world. Therapists work with the patients to uncover thoughts, beliefs, and images scarcely noticed. At its simplest, the patient asks, "What is going through my mind?" during a noticeable change in mood. Therapists and patients use several methods to elicit thoughts.

1.   Hot.—The best time to capture thoughts is when the emotions are intense. These thoughts are often most accessible as close to the triggering event as possible, when the patient is angry, sad, anxious, etc. The disadvantages are that the time may be inconvenient or the patient unable to write down thoughts.
2.   Cold.—Often, the more convenient time to write down thoughts is some time after the triggering event. The closer in time, the better. Time, circumstance, and mood may serve to cloud accurate memory for such "hot" cognitions. But what patients might lose in accuracy, they gain in convenience.
3.   Guided imagery.—Cognitions may be more accessible after allowing the patient to recreate the triggering event. The therapist guides the patient to recall the event in fine detail. The patient may then identify the sights, sounds, colors, textures, voices, noise, smells, temperature, tastes, etc. that characterize the image. Recall for the specific thoughts involved may be heightened after such an exercise.
4.   Induction.—The therapist can expose the patient to stimuli that trigger emotions and thoughts right in session. Such exposure plays a major role in the successful treatment of anxiety disorders. Overbreathing to induce hyperventilation and spinning to induce dizziness recreate feared physical sensations linked with

panic disorder. Similarly, reminders of loss can vividly trigger emotion-laden thoughts in the treatment of depression.

b. Questioning Thoughts. The main skills in cognitive therapy consist of the questioning of thoughts. Therapists ask questions and instruct patients to ask questions to help them examine their thoughts and mode of thinking. One mnemonic frequently used is FAST (Stephen McDermott, personal communication, Fall, 1991).

Facts: "Where's the evidence for this belief?" The therapist helps the patient examine the facts or evidence that back up their beliefs. If the patients' beliefs are like a tabletop, evidence forms the legs of that table. Patients use evidence, however biased or irrelevant, to support their beliefs. Newman (14) refers to three levels of evidence. 1) Conjectural evidence derives from intuition, without any observational proof: "I just know he doesn't like me, I can feel it"; 2) observational evidence rests on what one sees or hears: "I just know he doesn't like me, he sounded so rude"; 3) confirmational evidence is observational evidence easily confirmed by an objective third party: "I just know he doesn't like me, he said so." The patient works to find evidence that is confirmational, rather than purely observational or merely conjectural.

Alternatives: "What's another way to look at the evidence?" The therapist works with the patient to come up with alternative ways to look at the evidence for their beliefs. Patients hold biases about themselves and others. They may focus on evidence that is consistent with their biases, ignore evidence that is inconsistent, and distort evidence that is ambiguous. The search for alternatives allows patients to practice at some flexibility of thought and reframe their beliefs.

So what if it's true? This question has the patient examine the implications of their beliefs. This is comparable to what Ellis (15) refers to as the elegant or philosophical solution. The patient assumes that the belief is indeed true.

First, they ask themselves, "What's the worst that can happen?" Often, the worst is not as insurmountable as they might assume.

Next, they consider, "What's the best that can happen?" Often, they don't consider the best possibilities.

They then determine, "What's most likely to happen?" Often, the most realistic alternative is closer to the best alternative than to the worst.

Finally, they ask, "What constructively can I do?" The patient and therapist can work together to problem-solve. Jointly, they test possible solutions, decide upon a possible course of action, and make plans to carry it out.

Toll: Beliefs that patients hold have a price, but they also may point to an intended benefit. Patients can ask, "What's the effect of my thinking?" or "What disadvantages or costs does having this belief hold for me?" These beliefs, even if they hold more than a grain of truth, can demoralize or debilitate the patient. They can remove much of the fun and calm out of their lives.

In addition, patients may benefit from asking, "What are the advantages or benefits of having this belief?" Sometimes, the most painful beliefs may hide some potentially positive intent. Depressive beliefs may keep an individual from wasting precious energy in supposedly futile pursuits. Anxious beliefs may protect an individual from supposed harm. Acknowledging such intent can help the patient devise alternative methods to satisfy such intent. Patients can ask, "How can I increase the advantages and decrease the disadvantages of this belief?"

   c.   Cognitive Distortions.   The above questions provide guidelines to help the patient and therapist work together to examine problematic cognitions. In addition, it is often helpful for the patient and therapist to examine the specific cognitive distortions present in the patient's thinking. Labeling distortions can aid in correcting them.

Pointing out *all-or-none thinking* can help the patient look for and find the middle ground. A belief can change from "I failed the exam," to "Although I didn't meet my expectations, a B-minus is far from a failure."

Personalization/blame can help a patient look for multiple sources of responsibility and replace rumination with constructive action. "Who or what else might hold some measure of responsibility?"

Patients can examine *"should" statements* through questioning. 1) What are the advantages and disadvantages of telling myself, "I should . . ." 2) What constructive action can I take? 3) What are ways to reward myself for such action? 4) What rewards are inherent in doing it?

Magnification/minimization points to questioning the significance of the little events that trigger big feelings. "What's the meaning of this?'' or ''What bothers me most about this?'' The answers to such questions expose the added weight that magnifies seemingly trivial experiences. In addition, patients can minimize their qualities, talents, skills, abilities, and identity.

Labeling points out to the patients qualities in themselves and others that they gloss over with an unfair exaggeration. They can ask, ''What doesn't fit with this label?''

Mind reading/fortune telling points to the conclusions patients reach with limited information. They can question themselves to come up with alternatives, ''What else might he be thinking?'' or ''What else might happen?''

Emotional reasoning allows patients to determine if they are basing their beliefs on conjecture. They can learn to distinguish between feelings and facts by asking, ''Where is the evidence for this belief?'' They then can rely on evidence based on observation that can be objectively confirmed.

Mental filter allows the patient to note the positive details overshadowed by a single bit of negative information. Patients can ask, ''What piece of evidence may I be overlooking here?''

Overgeneralization points to patients' misuse of a single instance to hypothesize a general principle or pattern. They can ask, ''What contradicts this belief?''

Disqualifying the positive points to evidence that patients devalue or discount. They can question themselves to give proper consideration to positive information. They can ask, ''What information am I neglecting or not paying proper attention to?''

d. Behavioral Experiments. Patients can test the implications of their beliefs. For example, a person might expect rejection from others for holding the belief, ''If I disagree, they'll shun me.'' As preparation for assertiveness, the therapist can set up an experiment. The following steps can apply:

> *Specify the belief.* In what situations does this occur? If you do disagree, what happens? What hurts the most? What's the worst that can happen? The patient identifies the prediction, ''If I speak my mind, people will reject and ostracize me.''

Examine prior evidence. Who specifically rejected you? How long did they reject you? What were the circumstances? What areas of your life did this affect? How else can you look at this incident?

Set up an experiment. How can we test this? Therapist and patient devise a setting to test the belief, with maximum chances for safety and success.

Make predictions. The patient then makes predictions based on the old belief and predictions based on the alternative belief. The first prediction may be that people will ignore or attack what the patient says and reject him or her. The alternative prediction may be that they will listen to and consider what is said, and be accepting.

Examine the results. Therapist and patient examine how the results fit the predictions. What have you learned? What went right? What went wrong? What thoughts were going through your mind? In what way was your performance on target. In what ways could it improve? These questions can consolidate the learning and help plot future strategy and goals.

e. Core Beliefs Worksheet. After examining specific cognitions in specific situations, therapist and patient explore more general core beliefs. Feelings of despair in a variety of work situations could point to a core belief of incompetence. Feelings of despair in interactions with intimate others could reveal a core belief of unlovability. Either could relate to core beliefs of helplessness, powerlessness, lack of control, or defectiveness. The therapist helps patients expose these beliefs by asking for the meaning behind their most distressing feelings, thoughts, and triggers. The therapist and patient can follow these steps.

The patient identifies the core belief. A patient identifies the belief, "I'm incompetent." She then rates her strongest and weakest belief in it over the past week. If at some point belief is low, then the patient can note what alternative belief was held instead. If necessary, she and her therapist can devise a plausible alternative.

The patient then notes that alternative belief. She notes, "I'm competent in many areas. I have the ability to learn and to improve my performance." The patient then rates the strongest, weakest, and current belief in the alternative.

"Seek and ye shall find." The patient searches for evidence that supports the alternative. She gathers and records every bit of evidence that shows her ability to learn and demonstrates her competence.

The patient then records evidence that refutes the alternative, and adds a reframe. With such a reframe, the patient looks for alternative ways to look at the evidence. She can also plan constructive action to take despite the evidence.

The patient then rerates belief in the alternative. This exercise helps patients fight the tendency to overlook and distort evidence that disputes their biases.

3. Coping with the Emotional Component

Therapists can help patients deal with their emotions. They can help them accept emotions and encourage action in the face of emotional arousal. In depression, emotions can prompt patients to succumb to inactivity. They feel demoralized and do nothing rather than risk failure. They can magnify the meaning of emotions. They can make them a scourge, and signs of worthlessness, lack of control, or exclusion.

Cognitive therapy can help patients examine those beliefs about emotion that serve to add to the their distress. Such beliefs may develop out of parental models, early experiences, and family rules. They may survive because of the avoidance and the extremity of emotion that such beliefs help produce.

One model for dealing with the emotions is the AWARE model (16). It stands for Accept, Watch, Act With, Repeat the Above, and Expect the Best. Although designed for anxiety, this model works well with other emotions and even with ruminations.

Accept the emotion. Patients can treat emotion as a signal to act, not as an enemy. They can view it as important information to use, rather than as a transgression to condemn. For example, sadness may be a signal to examine and account for loss. Anxiety may be a signal to build and develop resources. Anger may signal time to review goals and problem-solve. Frustration may be a signal to measure strategies to surmount an obstacle. Patients can use the emotion, rather than catastrophize it.

Watch it. Patients can use several techniques to distance themselves from emotion. They can treat emotions scientifically, as one would measure, mark, and weigh matter. They can rate them on a scale from 1 to 10. Their attitude is to treat emotion as a potential good, worthy of examination. They can imagine what they would say to a friend with similar feelings. They can distract themselves from their emotions. They can focus their attention on people, or on a corner of a room, or the content of conversation.

Act with it. Emotion can be a signal to act, to problem-solve, to examine goals, to ask questions. Patients can view emotion not as a sign to stop, but as a sign to move.

Repeat the Above. Continue to accept, watch, and act with the emotion.

Expect the best. Eventually the emotion will lessen.

4. Suicidal Ideation

The major complication of depression is suicide. Individuals with a history of depression are more likely to attempt suicide. Alcohol and drug abuse are major risk factors for suicide. They impair rational thought and reduce inhibitions enough to make suicide an acceptable option. For these reasons, therapists must be alert to suicidal ideation and deal with it directly. When dealing with suicidal patients, the therapist can first assess whether the patient poses an immediate threat to his or her life. Hospitalization may protect patients in imminent danger. Otherwise, the following guidelines may be useful.

The therapist can assess the patient's reasons for living and dying. If possible, the therapist may encourage the patient to develop and add to the reasons for living. Therapist and patient can review prior reasons for living and determine if they do or can apply to the patient's life. They can also work together to help the patient come up with other reasons to choose life. The point is to help the patient tip the scales for living. This buys time and allows that critical period to pass without incident.

In addition, the therapist can help the patient examine for distortions the patient's reasons for dying. These often focus on death as an escape, as a means to solve problems that the patient regards as unsurmountable. Possible distortions: The patient may be unfairly labeling himself or herself as a loser because the problem has not as yet been solved. Partial solutions may be regarded as failures. A difficulty in one area of life may be generalized to all other areas as well. The therapist can attend to such distortions and help the patient respond to them. Therapists can assess other suicidal risk factors, such as previous attempts and suicidal thoughts, previous hospitalizations, and level of anxiety.

Other interventions work more towards prevention. Therapist, can encourage patients to seek the company of other concerned people. Therapists can instruct patients to avoid alcohol or drugs and to contact the therapist if any rough spots come. In addition, removing means and methods (guns, drugs) can reduce the ease and likelihood of suicidal gestures.

F. Summary

Depression is a risk for those in recovery from drug or alcohol abuse. In all stages of recovery, they are subject to the possibility of loss, to changes, risks, challenges, and relapse. For people prone to depression, such circumstances can trigger or exacerbate an episode. Depression, in turn, can be a trigger for relapse. This chapter has described a method for treatment of depression.

Cognitive therapy is more than a collection of techniques. It is a method to pull together information concerning a patient in emotional distress, set goals, and organize interventions. It provides a map for the planning and placement of treatment. It provides tools by which patients can cope with their own changes in mood and reduce this impact on their lives.

The cognitive model assumes that the inactivity and withdrawal associated with depression is brought on and encouraged by patients' beliefs. Hopelessness, a bleak world view, and low self-esteem combine to tell the patient, "What's the use? Why waste energy on fruitless pursuits?" Therapy helps depressed individuals examine such notions, test them for validity, and move beyond them. The therapist may initially provide the energy that the patients typically lack, but many times depressed patients underestimate their energies and abilities. Cognitive therapy helps patients to assess their abilities and take action. It helps patients reverse the pattern of passivity and withdrawal that fuels and validates depressive assumptions. Finally, cognitive therapy helps patients moderate moods that serve as both triggers and consequences of substance abuse. It initiates a cycle that can lead patients from relapse to recovery.

REFERENCES

1. A. T. Beck, A. J. Rush, B. F. Shaw, and G. Emery, *Cognitive Therapy of Depression,* Guilford Press, New York, 1979, pp. 1–33.

2. A. Freeman, and D. M. White, *Comprehensive Handbook of Cognitive Therapy* (A. Freeman, K. M. Simon, L. E. Beutler, and H. Arkowitz, eds.), Plenum Press, New York, 1989, p. 321.

3. A. T. Beck, F. D. Wright, C. F. Newman, and B. S. Liese, *Cognitive Therapy of Substance Abuse,* Guilford Press, New York, 1993, p. 12.

4. W. A. Hunt, L. W. Barnett, and L. G. Branch, *J. Clin. Psychol. 27:*455–456 (1971).

5. J. O. Prochaska, C. C. DiClemente, J. C. Norcross, *Am. Psychol. 47:*1102–1114 (1992).

6. D. D. Burns, *Feeling Good: The New Mood Therapy,* Signet, New York, 1981, p. 40.

7. A. T. Beck, *Arch. Gen. Psychiatry 41:*1112–1114 (1984).

8. M. E. P. Seligman, C. Castellon, J. Cacciola, P. Schulman, L. Luborsky, M. Ollove, and R. Downing, *J. Abnormal Psychol. 97:*13–18 (1988).

9. I. M. Blackburn, *Cognitive Psychotherapy: Theory and Practice* (C. Perris, I. M. Blackburn, and H. Perris, eds.), Springer-Verlag, Heidelberg, 1988, p. 98.

10. A. T. Beck, G. Brown, R. J. Berchick, B. Stewart, and R. A. Steer, *Am. J. Psychiatry 147:*190–195 (1990).

11. M. E. Weishaar, and A. T. Beck, *Int. Rev. Psychiatry 4:*177–184 (1992).

12. A. T. Beck, N. Epstein, G. Brown, and R. A. Steer, *J. Consult. Clin. Psychol.* 56(6):893–897 (1988).

13. A. T. Beck, C. H. Ward, M. Mendelson, J. Mock, and J. Erbaugh, *Arch. Gen. Psychiatry* 4:561–571 (1961).

14. C. F. Newman, The *Cognitive Behaviorist 10(3):*27–30 (1988).

15. A. Ellis, *Counseling Psychol.* 7:73–82 (1977).

16. A. T. Beck, G. Emery, and R. L. Greenberg, *Anxiety Disorders and Phobias: A Cognitive Perspective,* New York, 1985, pp. 323–324.

10

Interpersonal Psychotherapy

Sabrina Cherry
*Columbia University College of Physicians and Surgeons and
Presbyterian Hospital, New York, New York*

John C. Markowitz
Cornell University Medical College, New York, New York

I. INTRODUCTION

Interpersonal psychotherapy (IPT) was originally developed by Gerald Klerman and colleagues in the 1970s as a brief treatment for major depression (1). Since then, IPT has been adapted to treat specific subgroups of patients: depressed adolescent and geriatric patients (2,3), depressed HIV-infected patients (4), dysthymic patients (5), cocaine abusers (6,7), methadone-maintained opiate addicts (8), and patients with bulimia (9).

Practitioners of IPT use the connection between the patient's mood and his or her interaction with the social environment to help the patient find strategies that ameliorate both. By helping patients solve their difficulties with social roles, IPT both improves interpersonal functioning and treats the mood disorder.

Interpersonal psychotherapy has not been tested in the treatment of patients with alcohol use disorders. Although it might be used to help addicted patients achieve abstinence, their commitment to psychotherapeutic work is hindered by intoxication, withdrawal, and acute substance-related cognitive dysfunction. One of the only negative treatment trials of IPT was an attempt to apply it to cessation of cocaine use.

A strategy of more likely efficacy would be the adaptation of IPT to treat the interpersonal difficulties and dysphoria that substance-dependent patients experience after detoxification, in the early stages of rehabilitation. Faced with the havoc that chronic substance use has wreaked on their lives, relationships, and interpersonal and cognitive functioning, such patients are at high risk for relapse. With its medical model and its intuitively and emotionally reasonable approach to social functioning, IPT may be a comforting and helpful intervention for preserving early abstinence.

This chapter will present an overview of the practice of IPT for the treatment of depression and the research documenting its success. The original IPT format, which will be reviewed first, is applicable to alcoholics, whose recovery is often jeopardized by affective disorder (10–13). This chapter will then review studies in which IPT was adapted to treat opiate addicts and cocaine abusers; also, specific applications of IPT to the treatment of alcoholics in early recovery will be discussed.

II. OVERVIEW OF INTERPERSONAL PSYCHOTHERAPY

The theoretical roots of IPT arise from the work of Adolph Meyer and Harry Stack Sullivan (14,15). These clinical theorists emphasized the individual's connection to his social environment and the role of interpersonal relationships in the evolution and treatment of psychiatric disorders. Interpersonal psychotherapy emphasizes the patient's ongoing life circumstances and specifically examines the interactions between current situations and depression.

During IPT, the treatment of depression is focused in two main ways. First, following a medical model, the patient is told that he or she has a medical illness called depression and given the sick role. Second, one or more primary interpersonal problem areas are identified and linked to the depression. Sessions focus on recent life events and link these to affect. Affects and relationships are the principal focus, rather than cognitions as in cognitive therapy. Unlike psychoanalytic psychotherapy, IPT does not address transference, dream interpretation, or early childhood memories.

An IPT treatment usually consists of 12 to 20 weekly psychotherapy sessions lasting 50–60 minutes. Sessions are conducted by an experienced social worker, psychologist, or psychiatrist knowledgeable about the target disorder and with specific training in IPT. The therapist takes an active stance and at times guides the subject matter, ensuring that sessions stay on track. Therapists may make suggestions, encourage patients, and applaud their efforts when appropriate. The therapist allies with patients to help them choose among options and move toward higher functioning, more satisfying interpersonal relationships, and remission of depression.

A.   The Early Phase

Interpersonal psychotherapy can be broken into three phases: early (roughly sessions 1–3); middle (sessions 4–12); and late (sessions 13–16). The early phase establishes the basic alliance and treatment plan. Initially, this consists of diagnosing the depression according to Diagnostic and Statistical Manual (DSM)-IV criteria and quantifying the degree of depression using a rating scale such as the Hamilton Depression Rating Scale (16) or the Beck Depression Inventory (17). The rating scales can be used serially to track improvement later in treatment. The therapist should take a general psychiatric history to clarify whether additional diagnoses exist. Alternatives to outpatient IPT should be evaluated and consideration given to the concomitant use of medication, especially if the patient has a history of manic episodes, psychotic symptoms, severe personality disorders (particularly with profound social isolation or schizoid traits), or active self-destructive plans that may require more intensive treatment.

Once the diagnosis is established, the therapist elicits an Interpersonal Inventory to determine which interpersonal problem areas relate most closely to the current episode of depression. The Interpersonal Inventory is a review of key relationships, examining their quality of interactions, met and unmet expectations, patterns, and recent changes. Based on this, one of four interpersonal problem areas is usually chosen: grief, role dispute, role transition, or interpersonal deficit. The focus should be an area of difficulty that matches the patient's intuitive sense of the most pressing concerns, and upon which the patient and therapist agree.

With clarification of diagnosis and a focused interpersonal problem area, patients are offered an interpersonal formulation. First, patients should be told that they have a major depression and that this is a medical illness. Second, patients are given the "sick role"; that is, they are absolved of blame for being depressed and advised to take care of themselves including, when appropriate, getting assistance with or cutting back on daily responsibilities. At the same time, patients are instructed that an important responsibility of the sick role is to work in therapy towards recovery during the course of treatment (18). Third, the therapist links the interpersonal problem to the mood disturbance, and this linkage is suggested as the focus of treatment. Interpersonal psychotherapy avoids etiological assumptions about whether the interpersonal problem actually caused the depression or whether the depression led to the interpersonal problem. Factors are generally operating simultaneously by the time the patient seeks treatment. The following is an example of an interpersonal formulation within the problem area of a marital role dispute over infidelity.

> Your depression is linked to your dispute with your husband, whom you feel is still having an affair and not giving you the emotional attention you desire. Your guilty feelings, ruminations about your marriage, loss of interest in your social and family life, sleep difficulties, and hopelessness about the future should resolve as you address your feelings about your husband's infidelity and come to a resolution of your marital conflict. Your depression should lift as we focus on this issue during the next 3 months.

Another example of a formulation within the context of a role transition into parenthood is as follows.

> Your depression is related to the transition you are making from being a married professional to being a working parent. This transition has caused conflicts over balancing multiple demands, spending less time alone with your spouse, and developing parenting skills. As we discuss this transition in therapy and you make the most of the choices available to you, your sleep and appetite disturbance, feelings of despair, inadequacy, hopelessness, and anxiety should clear.

The formulation should be specific to the interpersonal problems as well as to the particular symptoms of depression.

B. The Middle Phase

The middle phase of IPT begins once the patient and the therapist have agreed on a diagnosis and interpersonal problem focus and contracted to spend the remainder of treatment addressing them. Sessions begin with the therapist asking the patient, "How have you been since we last met?" This question focuses the treatment in the "here and now" and elicits one of two responses. Usually, the patient will update progress in the interpersonal problem area, for example, whether they raised an issue with a spouse, or whether they tried a new social plan. If the patient reports such events, the therapist connects them to the patient's mood during this interval. Alternatively, the patient may describe his or her mood or depressive symptoms, which leads easily to further inquiry into events that may have influenced mood since the last session. In either case, the patient is helped to see the connection between mood and role or environment. Each interpersonal problem area has its own goals and strategies and will be outlined separately. Regardless of the problem area, patients are encouraged to make life improvements outside the sessions that increase activity and socialization. The increased activity counteracts the isolation that usually accompanies depression. Patients are encouraged to explore what they want in interpersonal situations and what options they can exercise to achieve their goals. The improved mood that usually follows these steps is highlighted in subsequent sessions.

1. Grief

Grief in and of itself is not a psychiatric disorder. Although features overlap with the classic symptoms of depression, the diagnosis of major depression is not made in the presence of uncomplicated bereavement. Grief may be abnormal if it is delayed or distorted. If a significant person in a patient's life has died and the patient appears not to have mourned the loss appropriately, grief should be considered as the focus of treatment. Abnormal grieving is suggested if patients have not experienced periods of sadness and loss after a death or if they have maintained a protracted active grieving state and have been unable to move on in their lives. Other clues that complicated bereavement may underlie a depressive episode include exacerbation around anniversaries of the death or of other, more recent losses. Guilty ruminations about the patient's relationship to the lost person, unresolved disputes, fantasies of joining the deceased, ongoing anxiety about not having prevented the death, and survivor guilt all suggest complicated bereavement (1).

The IPT strategy for treating complicated bereavement is to facilitate mourning and to help the patient find substitutes for the lost relationship. When grief is the problem area, the therapist encourages the patient to review his or her relationship with the deceased over time in both its good and bad aspects, clarifying the full range of feelings toward the individual, including unresolved disputes. This process should trigger feelings of normal grieving, including sadness, anger and loss. As this process unfolds, activities suggested by the therapist may stimulate grieving, such as visits to the grave, discussions with other family members, looking at pictures, or even organizing memorials to the lost individual.

Most important, however, is to provide a nonjudgmental, empathic environment in which patients can express their feelings. As grieving proceeds, it is appropriate to help the patient compensate for the loss by taking a new life course, whether that be socializing with friends, learning about finances, beginning to date, and so on. This final phase is central to the treatment of depression and may help with feelings of hopelessness, social withdrawal, and apathy.

For addicts in recovery, unresolved grief may have precipitated or exacerbated substance use. Feelings surrounding the original loss may resurface during abstinence. In addition, a death during the recovery period may increase relapse risk.

2. Role Disputes

The problem area of role disputes is chosen when the clearest precipitant of the patient's current depression is a conflict with a spouse, relative, close friend, or coworker. The cornerstone of role disputes is nonreciprocal expectations within a relationship that lead to an impasse (1). One potential scenario:

Mr. and Mrs. A have been married for 10 years, during which time Mr. A evolved the practice of regularly working overtime, eventually developing close relationships with coworkers that absorbed most of his emotional energy. Mrs. A felt lonely and angry home alone on evenings and weekends and unable to express her anger and loneliness to her husband. Despite making some new friends and enjoying her own work, she felt depressed, distanced from her husband, hopeless about her future, and suicidal. She sought treatment for depression.

Although this type of role dispute is fairly common, couples may be in different phases of addressing it when one partner seeks help. The couple might be aware of their differences and engaged in seeking solutions; emotionally distant, lacking awareness and communication skills; or in the midst of a complete breakdown of the relationship (1).

Interpersonal psychotherapy identifies the dispute, determines whether there is an impasse, and delineates the specific differences in expectations between the parties in a nonjudgmental manner. As in our example, we would first assess whether there is an impasse. Has our patient communicated to her husband her feelings about his schedule and its effect on their relationship? Has her husband responded, acknowledged the problem, or communicated his view? Is there ongoing dialogue regarding potential solutions? It is helpful to assess where in this process the impasse lies. Interventions encourage active discussion between the parties to break the impasse. The patient may gain insight into her own expectations and feelings about her husband's view. This phase may uncover feelings of anger, sadness, shame, or loss. As the patient actively engages with her husband and expresses her feelings, her depression is likely to lift, empowering her to take a more active role in conflict resolution. Having made explicit the differences between them and reduced the passivity of her depressive stance, the patient can then decide whether to compromise her own expectations, to assert her needs and ask her partner to change his pattern, or to choose another alternative, including ending the relationship. The therapist does not side with any choice, but supports the patient's active efforts toward conflict resolution, decision making, and attaining what she desires from the relationship. In sessions, the therapist emphasizes links between the patient's active efforts to resolve conflict at home and her improved affect.

For addicts in recovery, alcohol and drug use may have precipitated multiple role disputes around substance abuse behaviors that will need to be worked through during early recovery. In addition, substances may have been used to cope with long-standing role disputes and disappointments in a relationship that must be addressed in recovery to support abstinence.

3. Role Transition

The problem area of role transition is used when the depressed patient has recently undergone a change in a fundamental aspect of his or her life. Such transitions may include a change in job, living situation, or relationship, regardless of whether the change represents a success or a disappointment. Developmental changes such as becoming a parent, entering menopause, or aging may also precipitate depression. For an addict in recovery, abstinence itself is a role transition with multiple facets: accepting that drinking or drug use is a problem, entering a new social situation of abstinent friends, replacing substance use with other activities, and mending the damage that alcohol and drug behaviors have caused. Some patients may have initiated substance use to medicate premorbid anxiety, shyness, social awkwardness, and low self-confidence. These personality traits may resurface during abstinence and require new coping skills. Other patients may experience heightened dysphoria as a consequence of drinking or drug use and may need new skills in order to function.

Treatment within the context of a role transition involves mourning the loss of the old role and accepting the new one, acknowledging the positive and negative aspects of both roles and any anger and sadness accompanying the change. The therapist actively facilitates this process and encourages expression of affect related to the lost role. Labeling this period of flux a "role transition" for the patient and analyzing its connection to mood also provides a comforting framework in which to understand what the patient had experienced as chaos.

In addition to expressing feelings related to the loss of the old role, the patient is encouraged to take active steps toward adjusting to the new role and choosing among available options. This may include learning new skills, as in parenting, and seeking out support from others who have the needed skills. Alternatively, as in sobriety, active steps may include seeking out support and a social network in Alcoholics Anonymous (AA). Role playing in sessions can be used to facilitate this phase (1). As patients take active steps outside of sessions, their mood symptoms usually improve, hope is restored, and the patient feels more empowered in the new role.

4. Interpersonal Deficits

This final problem area of IPT should only be invoked if none of the other interpersonal problem areas apply. Patients in this category generally have characterologic problems leading to a paucity of relationships and minimal social supports. The therapist connects the depression to this lack of social connection or competence, and the treatment aims to reduce the patient's social isolation. This problem area fits less well into the short-term IPT model than the other categories, largely because it necessitates working with long-term character issues. This interpersonal problem area is the least well studied of the four and may include patients with worse prognoses (19).

Treatment consists of reviewing the positive and negative aspects of past and present relationships, searching for themes or trends. Such trends are then reviewed in the context of the patient's current relationships or, if none exist, of the relationship with the therapist. The latter relationship is treated as an example of a current relationship rather than as a manifestation of transference. Discussing feelings toward the therapist provides a model for communication and helps the patient learn how to negotiate relationships. The patient is encouraged to approach people to initiate relationships. Even contacts that result in less than happy outcomes are useful for the lessons they may then yield in therapy.

C. Termination Phase

As the last few sessions approach, the therapist reminds the patient of the anticipated termination date so that the patient is aware that they have entered the final phase of the process. The therapist's role in this phase is to outline the progress the patient has made and to reinforce the link between the resolution of depression and the steps the patient has taken in dealing with the interpersonal problem area. Rating scales can be repeated to quantify the extent of improvement and provide encouragement. If the patient has responded and depression has remitted, termination is a positive time: the steps the patient has taken to address problems are reviewed and posited as ways to deal with future problems or depressive symptoms that might arise. The competence developed in IPT empowers the patient to cope independently in the future. The therapeutic stance is supportive, encouraging, and optimistic about the patient's capacity to continue to use these new skills to maintain remission of symptoms.

Termination is also a time when sadness or anger may resurface in the transition out of therapy. In this context, symptoms may reemerge and can be dealt with in an open and encouraging manner. The patient is told that these feelings are a normal part of ending treatment and not necessarily a relapse of depression. A follow-up session scheduled 1 or 2 months later can be offered as reassurance and to allow the patient an opportunity to try new competencies on his own for a while. Termination may be the most difficult aspect of IPT for therapists trained in long-term psychotherapy, particularly if the patient has improved and the therapeutic alliance is strong. Therapists need to recall that the goal of IPT is to treat a target disorder, not to focus on long-term character issues.

If the patient has not responded to the therapy and is still significantly depressed, then this is a time to rethink the treatment plan. Was the diagnosis accurate? Were there intervening variables that sabotaged the treatment, such as ongoing substance abuse or too many missed sessions? Alternative treatments such as medication, a different therapist, or another mode of psychotherapy should also be considered. Particularly for depressed patients, it is important to counter their tendency to self-blame for the failure of treatment, and to reassure them that other treatment options exist.

D. Booster Sessions

We review below a study demonstrating the efficacy of monthly maintenance IPT in prophylaxis of recurrent depression. Depression is a recurrent illness, so continuation and maintenance therapy may often be a reasonable strategy. If monthly maintenance sessions are being considered, the end of the acute 16 week treatment should still be treated as a graduation with complete review of gains made. For the treatment of newly abstinent, vulnerable, alcohol-dependent patients, we anticipate that, should acute IPT be effective, maintenance sessions would be helpful for those making the transition to sobriety after years of drinking.

III. RESEARCH STUDIES OF INTERPERSONAL PSYCHOTHERAPY

The efficacy of IPT as an acute treatment for major depression has been established in two studies: the New Haven/Boston Collaborative Study of the Treatment of Acute Depression conducted by Klerman, Weissman, and colleagues (20–22) and the National Institute of Mental Health Treatment of Depression Collaborative Research Program (23,24).

A. The New Haven/Boston Study

The New Haven/Boston study was a controlled clinical trial carried out by Klerman, Weissman, and colleagues, begun in 1973, that studied 81 outpatients with unipolar, nonpsychotic major depression. Patients were randomized to receive 16-week treatments of amitriptyline alone, IPT alone, both IPT and amitriptyline, or a nonscheduled psychotherapy treatment. Treatment with amitriptyline consisted of doses of 125 mg daily by the first week, titration to doses between 100 mg and 200 mg daily by the third week, and then a stable dose for 12 weeks. Interpersonal psychotherapy consisted of 16 weekly 50-minute psychotherapy sessions according to the IPT manual (1). The nonscheduled treatment consisted of research interviews and assignment of patients to a psychiatrist whom they could contact and see a maximum of once a month.

Patients in all of the active treatments showed significantly lower treatment failure rates than those in the nonscheduled treatment. Combined treatment was more effective than either amitriptyline or IPT alone. Amitriptyline and IPT were equally effective, and each showed greater efficacy than the nonscheduled treatment (20).

The New Haven/Boston data revealed some differences in type of symptom reduction between amitriptyline and IPT. Patients receiving amitriptyline showed sleep improvement within 1 week, whereas improvement of anxiety, depression, and apathy took approximately 12 weeks. For patients receiving IPT, anxiety, depression, and apathy improved early, between weeks one and four. In both groups, the improvements were sustained throughout the 16 weeks. The authors concluded that medication had a rapid effect on vegetative symptoms, whereas IPT rapidly affected mood. There were no differential effects on social functioning (21).

A 1 year follow-up of the New Haven/Boston Study evaluated 62 of the 81 patients who received short term treatment for depression. Although most patients were doing well, many had received some form of subsequent treatment after the short-term study treatment ended. One differential long-term effect was found to correlate with initial treatment: patients who received IPT, with or without amitriptyline, reported significantly better social functioning, suggesting a later onset and lasting benefit of IPT in this area (22).

B. The National Institute of Mental Health Study

The National Institute for Mental Health (NIMH) Treatment of Depression Collaborative Research Program also documented the effectiveness of IPT as an acute treatment for major depression. This study, which excluded alcoholics, randomly assigned 250 patients with nonpsychotic, unipolar episodes of major depression to one of four 16-week treatments: cognitive behavioral therapy (CBT), as described by Beck and colleagues (25); interpersonal therapy (1); imipramine at doses averaging 185 mg per day with clinical management; and a pill-placebo condition, also with clinical management.

Analysis of those who completed treatment ($\geq$ 12 weeks) revealed treatment with imipramine to be most effective, whereas placebo was least effective. However, because the placebo/clinical management cell had a high response rate, no overall significant difference was found between treatments. The two psychotherapy groups had similar outcomes and an efficacy closer to imipramine than to placebo. The researchers stratified their results in *post hoc* analyses to compare outcomes of mildly depressed patients to those of more severely depressed patients. For mild depression (Ham-D < 20), there were no treatment differences. For more severely depressed patients (HAM-D ≥ 20), IPT was significantly superior to the placebo group on Hamilton Rating Scales and recovery criteria, and imipramine was superior to placebo on a wide range of measures. Cognitive behavioral therapy, however, did not show statistically significant superiority to placebo (23).

Sotsky and colleagues analyzed the NIMH data to establish whether patient characteristics might predict differential response to either IPT, CBT, or imipramine. Patients with less social dysfunction prior to treatment had better responses to IPT, whereas patients with less cognitive dysfunction responded better to CBT. Patients who were severely depressed and functionally impaired responded better to imipramine or IPT. Patients with high levels of work difficulties responded best to imipramine (24).

C. Interpersonal Psychotherapy as a Maintenance Treatment

One of the earliest IPT trials, also conducted as a collaborative New Haven/Boston study, assessed the efficacy of IPT and medication in preventing relapse of major depression. A total of 150 patients who were successfully treated with amitriptyline (100 to 200 mg/day) for 4 to 6 weeks were then randomized in a six-cell design to a maintenance phase and a follow-up phase of treatment. The cells included three medication groups: continuation of full-dose amitriptyline, a placebo group, and a no-pill group. The three medication groups were further randomized to two psychotherapy interventions: one cell received 1 hour of weekly psychotherapy (closely resembling IPT) and the other was a "low contact" group that saw psychiatrists for 15 minutes once a month for rating scales and drug management. Approximately 36% of those receiving no active medication or psychotherapy relapsed. Subjects receiving amitriptyline alone had a relapse rate of 12%, whereas those receiving IPT alone relapsed at a rate of 16.7%, not a statistically significant difference. There was no additive effect for the subset receiving combined treatment. However, IPT subjects did show a statistically significant improvement in measures of social adjustment that appeared 8 months into treatment (26). Further analysis delineated specific advantages for weekly IPT that peaked at approximately 8 months of follow-up: significantly less impaired work performance, fewer interpersonal disputes, improved communication skills, and less anxious rumination (27).

A more recent study of maintenance therapies for depression conducted in Pittsburgh confirmed the value of medication and IPT-M, a modified maintenance version of IPT, in long-term prophylaxis of recurrent major depression. Frank and colleagues followed up with patients during a 3-year period after successful treatment of an acute episode of major depression. These subjects had had at least three episodes of major depression and were thus at high risk for recurrence. The initial short-term treatment consisted of high-dose imipramine and weekly IPT. All responders then entered a 17-week continuation phase during which IPT sessions decreased to monthly frequency while medication was continued at full dose (mean > 200 mg/day). The 128 patients who continued symptom remission were randomized to combinations of maintenance high-dose medication and/or low-dose (monthly) psychotherapy. Treatment cells were: (1) IPT-M alone; (2) IPT-M and placebo; (3) IPT-M and imipramine; (4) medication clinic and placebo; and (5) medication clinic and imipramine. High-dose medication was the most effective prophylaxis with or without IPT-M, but IPT-M alone significantly delayed recurrence of depression. No significant interaction was noted when the two active treatments were combined, but there was a trend favoring combined treatment (28).

One analysis of the Pittsburgh data attempted to determine the specificity of IPT interventions in improving the length of symptom remission. Patient-therapist dyads able to keep a specifically interpersonal focus maintained significantly longer symptom remission compared with those dyads who veered from the IPT model (29).

D. Interpersonal Psychotherapy and Drug Abuse

Two studies of IPT have been conducted in substance abusing populations. One was conducted by Rounsaville and colleagues in a methadone program (8), the other by Carroll and colleagues in an outpatient treatment program for cocaine abusers (7), both in inner city New Haven.

In the methadone study, subjects were enrolled after completing the first 6 weeks in the methadone program, including the standard intensive initiation phase treatment of the New Haven program. Patients were eligible if they had comorbid axis I or axis II psychiatric disorders. Patients with antisocial personality disorder were included, whereas manic and schizophrenic patients were excluded from the study population. Seventy-two subjects were randomized to receive either IPT or a low contact treatment consisting of one 20-minute session per month with a psychiatrist. In addition, all subjects participated in the methadone program.

Of the 72 subjects randomized, 38% in the IPT cell and 54% of the low contact cell completed treatment. Most who left the IPT group withdrew voluntarily. Two subjects with ongoing substance use left the methadone program and two others had to be hospitalized for severe depression. The authors suggested that the low contact treatment had a lower attrition rate because less was demanded of these subjects to complete treatment.

Analysis of efficacy data showed little to suggest that IPT added benefit to the already intensive methadone program. It did not prove to be significantly more effective than the low contact treatment in reducing depression. This lack of apparent effect may have been because both groups improved, in part perhaps because the low contact group received group psychotherapy in the methadone program. The rich services received by the control group may have diminished the study's ability to show a benefit for IPT. Other administrative problems in study recruitment and retention may have affected outcome (8).

In a comparative trial to promote cocaine abstinence among outpatient cocaine abusers, IPT was no more and perhaps less effective than a behaviorally oriented treatment. Forty-two cocaine abusers were randomized to 12 weeks of either IPT or relapse prevention treatment (RPT), a treatment focused on reduction of drug craving and development of urge-coping strategies (30). Study subjects did not receive other treatments.

Twenty-four (55%) patients completed the study. The RPT group had less attrition throughout the study: by week twelve, the IPT dropout rate was twice that of RPT. Subjects assigned to RPT were more likely to achieve abstinence and be classified as symptomatically recovered, although these differences did not reach statistical significance. When data were stratified for severity of substance use and severity of psychiatric symptoms, RPT was significantly more effective than IPT in achieving abstinence among high-severity substance users (7).

Although these studies failed to demonstrate the efficacy of IPT in drug abusing populations, their results should not preclude applying IPT to early recovery in addicts. The cocaine study attempted to achieve abstinence while treating comorbid psychiatric pathology, a more complex task than that of the depression studies (31). In addition, the two drug abuse trials were conducted in inner city populations of substance abusers, burdened by multiple economic and social hardships. Finally, both trials included patients with antisocial personality disorder. This group has a poor prognosis and might reasonably be excluded from psychotherapy trials (12,13).

IV. INTERPERSONAL PSYCHOTHERAPY IN ALCOHOL RECOVERY

There are many potential uses for IPT during recovery from alcohol dependence. The model outlined in this chapter, based on Klerman and colleagues' original application of IPT for depression, can be implemented with the significant subgroup of alcoholics in recovery who suffer from major depression or dysthymia. Also, IPT can be adapted to focus on the abstinence period regardless of whether a mood disorder is present. The cocaine abuse study by Carroll and colleagues used a version of IPT specifically adapted for cocaine use that attempted to incorporate abstinence concepts into the standard IPT model. This involved focusing on three goals in addition to the interpersonal problem area: acceptance of the need to stop, management of impulsiveness, and recognition of the context of drug use and supply (6). A similar adaptation of IPT for alcohol dependent patients in early abstinence (IPT-EAA) is being developed by Markowitz and colleagues at Cornell University Medical College/New York Hospital-Westchester Division in White Plains, New York. As has been the case in other adaptations of IPT, a manual modifying IPT to meet the specific psychosocial needs of this population will be developed.

Research on recovery from alcohol dependence indicates the role of interpersonal functioning as a key prognostic indicator. Two separate longitudinal studies have shown the importance of social and work relationships as a factor in recovery. Vaillant's study of 400 inner city men found that the acquisition of a new close relationship was associated with successful first year abstinence (32). Another prospective study conducted in Sweden showed that alcoholics with a greater prevalence of family problems, greater interpersonal isolation, and greater isolation and exclusion from the labor market had poorer prognoses. Good prognostic indicators included emotional and social stability and satisfaction in work and interpersonal relationships (33).

Studies of relapse prevention also suggest that interpersonal problems predict relapse. In addition to intrapersonal factors (i.e. positive and negative emotional states), such interpersonal factors as relationship conflict, social pressure to use substances, lack of family support, lack of productive work roles, and lack of involvement in leisure or recreational activity all predict higher relapse rates (34–36). Stressful life events, such as legal or economic problems or the death of a close friend, were found to be more common among relapsed alcoholics than among recovered patients or community controls (37). The same study showed that family functioning was also poorer among relapsed alcoholics (38). In a study by Finney and colleagues, the number of negative life events during the first 6 months of abstinence predicted treatment outcome at 2-year follow-up (39). In addition, relapsed alcoholics showed less self confidence, less ambition, and less outgoing behavior after relapse compared with abstinent alcoholics and community controls (37). Moos and Finney conclude that addressing patients' ongoing life circumstances would make alcoholism treatment more effective (36).

These studies of prognosis and relapse prevention suggest that addressing a patient's current interpersonal functioning should be a central component of treatment during recovery from alcohol dependence. The focus of IPT on a current relationship dispute, a role transition, death of a loved one, or an interpersonal deficit targets these aspects of recovery. Specifically, role disputes within a marriage or at work may predate drinking or become enmeshed with behaviors induced by alcohol, such as impulsivity, aggression, or irresponsibility. Becoming sober constitutes a role transition where social skill deficits may resurface. As Nakamura and colleagues noted, individuals whose social adjustment depended on alcohol are at greater risk for depression in recovery (40). Given its success in treating the interpersonal difficulties of patients with depression and other disorders (41), IPT may be adapted and applied to the interpersonal problems of alcoholic patients in early abstinence with a clear potential to enhance outcome.

In addition, IPT might be effective when combined with medication. O'Malley and colleagues combined naltrexone with either coping skills/ RPT or supportive psychotherapy and found that subjects taking naltrexone and receiving supportive psychotherapy were less likely to resume drinking (42). The foundation of IPT in the medical model facilitates its use in conjunction with pharmacologic treatments.

Multiple treatments have already targeted the psychosocial problems that alcoholics face in recovery, including individual psychodynamic and behavioral therapies, group therapy, family therapy, and AA (43,44). More recently, interactional group therapy (45–47) has been studied, as have cognitive-behavioral therapies (48), including coping skills/relapse prevention (30), social skills training (49), and relaxation training (50). Although many of these treatments have shown promise within subgroups, no treatment has been consistently efficacious in preventing relapse (43). As outlined in this chapter, IPT distinctly differs from these cognitive/behavioral treatments in its focus on the connection between mood and events in the patient's life and relationships. Although its efficacy in alcohol recovery is as yet undocumented, its orientation might fill a niche in the repertoire of available treatments.

REFERENCES

1. G. L. Klerman, M. M. Weissman, B. J. Rounsaville, and E. S. Chevron, *Interpersonal Psychotherapy of Depression* Basic Books, New York (1984), pp. 73–142.
2. D. Moreau, L. Mufson, M. M. Weissman, and G. L. Klerman, *J. Am. Acad. Child Adolesc. Psychiatry 30:*642–651 (1991).
3. E. Frank, N. Frank, C. Cornes, S. D. Imber, M. Miller, S. Morris, and C. F. Reynolds, *New Applications of Interpersonal Psychotherapy* (G. Klerman and M. Weissman, eds.), American Psychiatric Press, Washington, D.C., 1993, p. 167.

4. J. C. Markowitz, G. L. Klerman, and S. W. Perry, *Hospital and Community Psychiatry 43:*885 (1992).

5. B. J. Mason, J. C. Markowitz, and G. L. Klerman, *New Applications of Interpersonal Psychotherapy* (G. Klerman and M. Weissman, eds.), American Psychiatric Press, Washington, D.C., 1993, p. 225–264.

6. B. J. Rounsaville, F. Gawin, and H. Kleber, *Am. J. Drug Alcohol Abuse 11:*171 (1985).

7. K. M. Carroll, B. J. Rounsaville, and F. H. Gawin, *Am. J. Drug Alcohol Abuse 17:*229 (1991).

8. B. J. Rounsaville, W. Glazer, C. H. Wilber, M. M. Weissman, and H. D. Kleber, *Arch. Gen. Psychiatry 40:*629 (1983).

9. C. G. Fairburn, R. Jones, R. C. Peveler, S. J. Carr, R. A. Solomon, M. E. O'Connor, J. Burton, and R. A. Hope, *Arch. Gen. Psychiatry 48:*463 (1991).

10. R. Cadoret, and G. Winokur, *Ann. N. Y. Acad. of Sciences 233:*34 (1974).

11. D. Behar, G. Winokur, and C. J. Berg, *Am. J. Psychiatry 141:*1105 (1984).

12. A. T. McLellan, L. Luborsky, G. Woody, C. P. O'Brien, and K. A. Druley, *Arch. Gen. Psychiatry 40:*620 (1983).

13. B. J. Rounsaville, Z. S. Dolinsky, T. F. Babor, and R. E. Meyer, *Arch. Gen. Psychiatry 44:*505 (1986).

14. A. Meyer, *Psychobiology: A Science of Man,* Charles C. Thomas, Illinois, 1957.

15. H. S. Sullivan, *The Interpersonal Theory of Psychiatry,* W. W. Norton, New York, 1953, pp. 3–45.

16. M. Hamilton. *J Neurol Neurosurg Psychiatry, 25:*56 (1960).

17. A. T. Beck, C. Ward, and M. Mendelson, *Arch. Gen. Psychiatry 42:*667 (1961).

18. T. Parsons, *Am. J. Orthopsychiatry 21:*452 (1951).

19. J. C. Markowitz, and M. M. Weissman, *Handbook of Depression,* (E. E. Beckham, and W. R. Leber, eds., Second Edition), Guilford, New York, (in press).

20. M. M. Weissman, B. A. Prusoff, A. DiMascio, C. Neu, M. Goklaney, and G. L. Klerman, *Am. J. Psychiatry 136:*555 (1979).

21. A. DiMascio, M. M. Weissman, B. A. Prusoff, C. Neu, M. Zwilling, and G. L. Klerman, *Arch. Gen. Psychiatry 36:*1450 (1979).

22. M. M. Weissman, G. L. Klerman, B. A. Prusoff, D. Sholomskas, and N. Padian, *Arch. Gen. Psychiatry 38:*51 (1981).

23. I. Elkin, T. Shea, J. T. Watkins, S. D. Imber, S. M. Sotsky, J. F. Collins, D. R. Glass, P. A. Pilkonis, W. R. Leber, J. P. Docherty, S. J. Fiester, and M. B. Parloff, *Arch. Gen. Psychiatry 46:*971 (1989).

24. S. M. Sotsky, D. R. Glass, M. T. Shea, P. A. Pilkonis, J. F. Collins, I.
     Elkin, J. T. Watkins, S. D. Imber, W. R. Leber, J. Moyer, M. E. Oliveri,
     *Am. J. Psychiatry 148:*997 (1991).

25. A. T. Beck, A. J. Rush, B. F. Shaw, and G. Emery, *Cognitive Therapy
     of Depression,* Guilford, New York, 1979, pp. 1–34.

26. G. L. Klerman, A. DiMascio, M. M. Weissman, B. Prusoff, E. Paykill,
     Am. J. Psychiatry 131: 186 (1974).

27. M. M. Weissman, G. L. Klerman, E. S. Paykill, B. Prusoff, and B.
     Hanson, *Arch. Gen. Psychiatry 30:*771 (1974).

28. E. Frank, D. J. Kupfer, J. M. Perel, C. Cornes, D. B. Jarrett, A. Mallinger,
     M. E. Thase, A. B. McEachran, and V. J. Grochocinski, *Arch. Gen.
     Psychiatry 47:*1093 (1990).

29. E. Frank, D. J. Kupfer, E. F. Wagner, A. B. McEachran, and C. Cornes,
     *Arch. Gen. Psychiatry 48:*1053 (1991).

30. G. A. Marlatt and J. R. Gordon, *Relapse Prevention,* Guilford, New
     York, 1985, p. 3–124.

31. B. J. Rounsaville and K. Carroll, *New Applications of Interpersonal
     Psychotherapy* (G. Klerman, and M. Weissman, eds.), American Psychi-
     atric Press, Washington D.C., 1993, pp. 319–353.

32. G. E. Vaillant and E. S. Milofsky, *Arch. Gen. Psychiatry 39:*127 (1982).

33. S. Ojesjo, *Br. J. Addiction 76:*391 (1981).

34. K. Bronwell, G. A. Marlatt, E. Lichtenstein, and G. T. Wilson, *Am.
     Psychologist 41:*765 (1986).

35. D. Daley and G. A. Marlatt, *Substance Abuse: A Comprehensive Text-
     book,* (J. Lowinson, P. Ruiz, and R. B. Millman, eds.), Williams and
     Wilkins, Baltimore, 1992, pp. 533–543.

36. R. H. Moos and J. W. Finney, *Am. Psychologist 38:*1036 (1983).

37. R. H. Moos, J. W. Finney, and D. A. Chan, *J. Stud. Alcohol 42:*383
     (1981).

38. R. H. Moos and B. S. Moos, *J. Stud. Alcohol 45:*111 (1984).

39. J. W. Finney, R. H. Moos, and C. R. Mewborn, *J. Consult. Clin. Psychol.
     48:*17 (1980).

40. M. M. Nakamura, J. E. Overall, L. E. Hollista, and E. Radcliffe, *Alcohol-
     ism: Clin. Exp. Res. 7:*188 (1983).

41. G. Klerman and M. M. Weissman, *New Applications of Interpersonal
     Psychotherapy* (G. Klerman and M. Weissman, eds.), American Psychiat-
     ric Press, Washington, D.C., 1993, pp. 27–51.

42. S. S. O'Malley, A. J. Jaffe, G. Chang, R. Schottenfeld, R. E. Meyer,
     and B. Rounsaville, *Arch. Gen. Psychiatry 49:*881 (1992).

43. *Prevention and Treatment of Alcohol Problems: Research Opportunities*

(Institute of Medicine, ed.), National Academy Press, Washington D.C., 1989.

44. R. K. Hester, and W. R. Miller, *Handbook of Alcoholism Treatment Approaches,* New York, 1989, pp. 1–292.

45. S. Brown, and I. Yalom, *J. Stud. Alcohol. 38:*426 (1977).

46. R. M. Kadden, N. L. Cooney, H. Getter, and M. D. Litt, *J. Consult. Clin. Psychology, 57:*698 (1989).

47. N. L. Cooney, R. M. Kadden, M. D. Litt, H. Getter, *J. Consult. Clin. Psychol. 59:*598 (1991).

48. D. W. Foy, L. B. Nunn, and R. G. Rychtarik, *J. Consult. Clin. Psychol. 52:*218 (1984).

49. E. F. Chaney, M. R. O'Leary, and G. A. Marlatt, *J. Consult. Clin. Psychol. 46:*1092 (1978).

50. F. Klajner, L. M. Hartman, M. B. Sobell, *Addictive Behaviors 9:*41 (1984).

11

Problem-Solving Therapy

Arthur M. Nezu, Christine Maguth Nezu, and Jami L. Rothenberg
Medical College of Pennsylvania and Hahnemann University, Philadelphia, Pennsylvania

Thomas J. D'Zurilla
State University of New York at Stony Brook, Stony Brook, New York

I. INTRODUCTION

Interest and empirical scrutiny addressing the construct of problem solving in humans has a long and full history. It has been only recently, however, that mental health professionals have focused on this construct as a way to understand its role in the etiopathogenesis and treatment of various behavioral disorders and emotional problems. At present, problem-solving therapy continues to gain support as an effective clinical intervention in a variety of psychological disorders, including depression (1). Our approach to this form of therapy is based heavily on the conceptual model of social problem solving originally articulated by D'Zurilla and Goldfried (2) and later revised by D'Zurilla and Nezu (3). We begin this chapter with a set of definitions regarding our model of social problem-solving training. Problem-solving assessment strategies are described next, followed by a brief review of the empirical literature regarding problem-solving training for both depression and substance abuse. The remainder of the chapter includes an abbreviated "treatment manual" that can serve as a guide to clinicians who wish to apply this intervention to patients experiencing depression during the recovery process.

A. Social Problem Solving Defined

We have previously defined social problem solving as the metacognitive process by which individuals understand the nature of problems in living and direct their attempts to altering either (a) the problematic nature of the situation itself, (b) their reactions to them, or (c) both (4,5). Problems are defined within our approach as specific life situations (either present or anticipated) that demand responses for adaptive functioning but do not receive effective coping responses from the individuals confronted with them because of the presence of various obstacles. Such obstacles may include ambiguity, uncertainty, conflicting demands, lack of resources, and/or novelty.

Essentially, problems often represent a discrepancy between the reality of a situation and one's desired goals (4,5). Problems are likely to be stressful if they are at all difficult or relevant to well being (6). A problem can be a single event (for example, missing a train to work), a series of related events (such as difficulties with a coworker), or a chronic situation (such as a distressed marital relationship). The demands in the problematic situation can originate in one's interpersonal environment (lack of job opportunities, an argument with a parent) or within the person him or herself (personal goal, need, commitment).

According to our definition, a problem is not a characteristic of either the environment or person alone. Rather, a problem is a particular type of person-environment relation that reflects a perceived imbalance or discrepancy between demands and adaptive response availability. This imbalance is likely to change over time, depending on changes in the environment, the person, or both.

In our model, a solution is defined as any coping response designed to alter the nature of the problematic situation, one's negative emotional reactions to it, or both (1). Effective solutions are those coping responses that not only achieve these goals, but simultaneously maximize other positive effects and minimize negative effects (3). These associated benefits and costs involve the short- and long-term implications of a solution, as well as both the personal consequences for the individual and the impact that the solution has on significant others. The adequacy or effectiveness of any potential solution varies from person to person and from setting to setting because the perceived effectiveness of a particular problem-solving response also depends on one's values, goals, or significant others.

Problem-solving capacity can be further characterized as consisting of a series of specific skills rather than a single unitary ability. According to D'Zurilla and Nezu (3), effective problem solving requires five interacting component processes, each of which makes a distinct contribution to effective problem resolution. These processes are problem orientation, problem definition and formulation, generation of alternatives, decision making, and solution implementation and verification.

The problem-orientation component differs from the other four components in that it is a motivational process, whereas the other components consist of specific skills and abilities that enable a person to solve a particular problem effectively. Problem orientation can be described as a set of orienting responses representing the immediate cognitive-affective-behavioral reactions of a person when first confronted with a problematic situation. These orienting responses include a general sensitivity to problems, as well as various beliefs, assumptions, appraisals, and expectations concerning life's problems and one's own problem-solving ability. This psychological set is based primarily on a person's developmental and reinforcement history related to real-life problem solving. Depending on the specific nature of these variables, one's orientation can engender positive affect and approach motivation, in turn facilitating effective problem solving, or it might lead to negative affect and avoidance motivation, which can inhibit or disrupt subsequent problem-solving attempts.

The remaining four components of the problem-solving process constitute a set of specific skills or goal-directed tasks that enable a person to solve a particular problem successfully. Each task makes a distinct contribution toward the discovery of an adaptive solution or coping response in a problem-solving situation. The goal of problem definition and formulation is to clarify and understand the specific nature of the problem, as well as to specify a set of realistic goals and objectives. The purpose of the third task, generation of alternatives, is to list via brainstorming techniques as many solutions as possible to increase the likelihood that the most effective ideas will be offered. The goal of decision-making is to conduct a cost-benefit analysis concerning each solution alternative and to apply the best one(s) to the actual problem situation. Finally, the purpose of solution implementation and verification is to monitor and evaluate the effectiveness of the implemented solution, as well as to troubleshoot if the outcome is unsatisfactory.

These five processes are not based on a natural classification of cognitive-behavioral strategies used by individuals in the real world. Rather, they represent a pragmatic format for training individuals in effective problem resolution and coping. The sequence specified above, however, does not imply that such problem solving should proceed in a unidirectional fashion. Instead, effective problem solving is likely to involve continuous movement among the five components before a problem is satisfactorily resolved, especially if it is complex. For example, while attempting to make decisions, a person may realize that he or she did not generate a sufficient number of solution ideas. In such cases, a return to that task may be necessary before a selection is made.

There are two major reasons why people may have difficulty effectively resolving problems in living. First, the person may not have learned the necessary problem-solving skills. Second, the individual may have acquired these skills, but may fail to demonstrate effective problem solving in a particular situation because of negative emotions, such as anxiety or depression, that inhibit the performance of any or all of the various problem-solving operations. Training in both cases should be helpful.

II. PROBLEM-SOLVING ASSESSMENT

Assessment of a person's overall problem-solving competence should focus on both his or her problem-solving *ability* and *performance*. Ability refers to the knowledge and understanding of various critical problem-solving processes, whereas performance reflects the application of this knowledge to a particular real-life problem. Although it is likely that these two problem-solving variables are related, clinical evaluation of both becomes important when identifying specific deficits and idiosyncratic problem areas. For instance, a person may be able to generate a wide range of alternative solutions to a problem but may experience difficulty in inhibiting the impulsive implementation of a solution. Treatment for such an individual would concentrate more on enhancing his or her problem-solving performance skills rather than on practicing brainstorming techniques.

A comprehensive discussion of certain theoretical and psychometric issues surrounding problem-solving assessment is far beyond the scope of this chapter (the interested reader is referred elsewhere [3,7] for such information). Therefore, we will limit our discussion here to descriptions of certain popular measures of problem solving that can be useful to clinicians working with adults.

Assessment of a patient's problem-solving competence can involve several different formats: (a) self-report inventories, (b) paper-and-pencil performance tasks, and (c) structured interviews and role plays.

Two popular self-report questionnaires include the Problem-Solving Inventory (PSI) (8) and the revised version of the Social Problem-Solving Inventory (SPSI-R) (9,10). The PSI is a 32-item Likert-type questionnaire that measures a person's problem-solving self-appraisal, that is, an individual's perceptions and self-evaluations of his or her own problem-solving behavior and attitudes. This inventory was originally developed based on the D'Zurilla and Goldfried (2) five-component model. A factor analysis of an initial 50-item pool led to the identification of three distinct factors: (a) problem-solving confidence (belief and trust in one's problem-solving abilities); (b) approach-avoidance style (general tendency to approach or avoid different problem-solving activities); and (c) personal control (beliefs concerning one's self-control over emotions and behaviors during problem solving). The most popular PSI measure has been the total score, but three scale scores corresponding to these three factors can also be obtained from the 32 items.

The original SPSI (10) was a 70-item Likert-type self-report measure of social problem-solving ability directly based on the D'Zurilla and Nezu (3) conceptual model. More recently, the SPSI was revised based on a principal axes factor analysis (9). The resulting inventory, the

SPSI-R, now contains 52 items within five unidimensional scales: (a) *Positive Problem Orientation* (a cognitive set reflecting an adaptive, facilitative approach); (b) *Negative Problem Orientation* (inhibitive and disruptive cognitive processes and emotional states); (c) *Rational Problem Solving* (the rational and systematic application of effective problem-solving principles and techniques; includes subscales reflective of the four problem-solving tasks of problem definition and formulation, generation of alternatives, decision making, and solution implementation and verification); (d) *Impulsivity/Carelessness Style* (an impulsive and careless problem-solving style); and (e) *Avoidance Scale* (a problem-solving style reflecting procrastination, passivity, and dependency).

Because both the PSI and SPSI have been used in research studies evaluating the effects of problem-solving therapy for depression and have been found to be sensitive to changes occurring as a function of such training (11–13), clinicians can use these inventories to measure improvement in their patients.

The Means-End Problem-Solving (MEPS) procedure (14) is an example of a problem-solving outcome measure. Outcome measures focus on the quality of the output or end result of the problem-solving process—the solution. In the MEPS procedure, subjects are presented with a series of 10 hypothetical interpersonal problems or conflict situations consisting of incomplete stories that only have a beginning and an ending. In the beginning of the story, the need or goal of the protagonist is specified (for example, the desire to make new friends), and, at the end of the story, the protagonist successfully satisfies that need or achieves the goal (actually makes new friends). Subjects are asked to articulate the means by which the protagonist gets from ''A'' to ''B,'' that is, how the person achieves the goal specified in the story.

Additional methods of assessing a patient's problem-solving ability involve the use of structured interviews and role playing of hypothetical problem situations (3,15). The therapist's observation of a patient's abilities and performance can occur during discussions of actual problems. Also, patients can be asked to keep a diary or record of various problems and their attempts in solving those that may occur between sessions (see [1,4] for sample forms).

III. PROBLEM SOLVING AND DEPRESSION

Recently, Nezu, Nezu and Perri (1,5) have articulated a model of unipolar depression that identifies deficits in problem-solving as a significant vulnerability factor. Briefly put, when deficits in problem-solving skills lead to ineffective coping attempts under high levels of stress (emanating either from major negative life events or from continuous daily problems or "hassles"), depression is likely to ensue (1,5). Support for this conceptualization draws upon several sources of empirical investigations.

One group of studies points to the significant association between ineffective problem-solving ability and level of depressive symptomatology. Gotlib and Asarnow (16), for example, found that a sample of depressed college students performed less effectively on the MEPS than a nondepressed control group. In addition, Nezu and Ronan (17) evaluated differences between depressed and nondepressed college students regarding their ability to generate alternatives to a series of real-life problems. Results indicated that the depressed subjects produced solutions that were rated as being significantly less effective than those of nondepressed subjects. In addition, the depressed individuals generated significantly fewer alternatives than their nondepressed counterparts. More importantly, these authors found that training in this skill ameliorated this depression-related deficit. In a related second study, similar results were found with regard to decision-making ability (17). Specifically, depressed subjects, when offered a wide range of alternative solutions to a series of interpersonal, real-life problems, were found to choose less effective alternatives compared with nondepressed controls. However, as in the previous study, training in decision making was found to facilitate better performance for both the depressed and nondepressed subjects.

Additional research has incorporated the PSI (8) to assess the relation between problem solving and depression. Nezu (18), for example, used the PSI to distinguish between "ineffective problem solvers" and "effective problem solvers" and found that effective problem solvers reported significantly lower Beck Depression Inventory (BDI) scores (19) than ineffective problem solvers. Ineffective problem solvers have also been found to report significantly higher scores on the depression scale of the Minnesota Multiphasic Personality Inventory (MMPI) relative to effective problem solvers (20).

Because many of the above studies focused exclusively on depression-related deficits in problem solving among college students or subclinical populations, Nezu (21) conducted a further investigation that involved clinically depressed individuals. Depressed individuals were identified as those who had received a diagnosis of major depressive disorder according to criteria outlined by the Diagnostic and Statistical Manual (22). Results indicated that depressed subjects were characterized by problem-solving deficits when compared with the nondepressed controls.

Marx, Williams, and Claridge (23) also focused on a population of reliably diagnosed, clinically depressed patients and found additional evidence of a deficit in social problem solving in such individuals. Depressed subjects displayed difficulties in solving hypothetical and personal problems and reported negative attitudes toward problems and problem solving.

Consistent with these findings are two additional studies. Doerfler and Richards (24) examined differences between adult women who were successful and unsuccessful in self-initiated attempts to cope with depressive episodes. Successful women were found to have engaged in more effective problem-solving attempts to overcome their depression. Beckham and Adams (25) conducted a similar study with 164 clinically depressed individuals and found converging results. Specifically, subjects indicated that they viewed ''taking action on problems'' as one of the most helpful strategies for feeling better.

A second group of studies have conceptualized problem-solving skills as a potential buffer or moderator of the negative effects of life stress. For example, Nezu and Ronan (26) proposed a causal model that incorporated negative life stress, current problems, problem-solving coping, and depressive symptomatology. Using path analytic techniques, results from a study involving 205 subjects provided strong support for the following relations among these variables: (1) experiencing negative stressful events results in an increase in problematic situations; (2) the degree to which individuals effectively cope with these problems is a function of their problem-solving ability; and (3) effective resolution of these problems serves to decrease the probability of depressive symptoms.

An illustration of this model might involve the individual who gets fired from his job. According to the early literature on life-change events, this situation would have been considered a major negative event and the only definition of the construct of stress measured. However, Nezu and Ronan (26) suggested that as a consequence of such an event, additional related problems might occur, such as finding a new job, managing daily finances, and identifying ways to use the newly increased free time. These related problems serve as additional sources of stress beyond the event itself. Further, even if the problem of obtaining new employment can be readily solved, adjustment to the new position creates its own series of problems, such as finding new transportation routes or dealing with new supervisors. Thus, the authors posited that effective resolution of this wide range of problems serves to decrease the probability of the individual experiencing depression. Conversely, ineffective problem-solving coping would make the individual more vulnerable to a depressive episode. With regard to the depression-engendering nature of stressful problems, Nezu (27) found that assessment of life events and current problems each predicted a level of depressive symptoms, but the influence of both sources combined was greater and a better predictor than either variable considered alone. Further support for the significant stress-buffering function of problem solving is provided by several additional studies (28–30).

An important corollary of the problem-solving model of depression implies that training in these skills should lead to decreases in overall distress and increases in overall coping (1,5). Furthermore, it is hypothesized that problem-solving training will foster an individual's ability to effectively and independently cope with new problems once training has concluded (1). These populations have gained increasing support from well-controlled studies that document problem-solving training to be highly efficacious as a treatment for clinical depression in middle-aged adults (11,12), adults with mental retardation (31), and elderly adults (13,32). Of particular importance is the consistent finding that the positive effects of problem-solving treatment, such as a decrease in depression and an increase in coping skills, is maintained over time (11,12).

IV. PROBLEM SOLVING AND SUBSTANCE ABUSE

Researchers have also addressed the relation between problem-solving skills and addictive disorders—alcoholism in particular. This is based on the hypothesis that for abusers, alcohol often is the chosen ''solution'' for dealing with negative feelings and problems (33). In other words, individuals who abuse alcohol may not have the ability to generate alternative solutions to cope with life's difficulties (34). For example, Williams and Kleinfelter (35) investigated alcohol use in a college population and found that students with lower confidence in problem-solving capabilities reported greater use of alcohol to cope with negative emotions and to escape from responsibilities than students with high confidence in their abilities. In addition, Carey and Carey (36) found a population of dually-diagnosed psychiatric patients to have significantly poorer social problem-solving skills than community controls. Nixon and colleagues (37) further found that both female and male adult alcoholics exhibited similar interpersonal problem-solving deficits when compared with controls.

Investigators have also used problem-solving training as a means of promoting behavior change in abusers. For example, Intagliatia (38) conducted a controlled treatment outcome study evaluating the efficacy of problem-solving training. Those subjects who participated in a problem-solving protocol, in addition to receiving standard hospital care for alcoholism, performed significantly better than controls with regard to their ability to plan and prepare for coping with problems in living after returning to the community.

In a more recent study, recovering alcoholics receiving problem-solving training were found to report fewer relapses and drinking-related problems when compared with controls (39). Platt et al. (34) also found that training in problem solving was successful in reducing problematic behaviors for both incarcerated heroin addicts and alcoholics.

Problem-solving training begun at an early age has also been shown to be useful in reducing the risk of abusing alcohol as a coping mechanism in dealing with difficult situations. Elias and colleagues (40) implemented a 2-year social problem-solving training program for elementary school students. Those receiving the training were found to demonstrate higher levels of prosocial behaviors and lower levels of antisocial and self-destructive behaviors when followed up in high school 4–6 years later, compared with controls. This research team also found that boys who did not receive training were characterized by higher levels of self-destructive and alcohol-related behaviors, whereas girls were involved more often with tobacco use.

In sum, substantial research has pointed to a strong relation between problem-solving deficits and both depression and substance abuse. More importantly, research has also documented the efficacy of a problem-solving approach to clinical intervention with these populations. The remainder of this chapter will provide a brief "therapy manual" to guide clinicians in applying problem-solving therapy for depression.

V. SOCIAL PROBLEM-SOLVING TRAINING

A. Treatment Goals

The goals of our approach to problem-solving therapy in general include: (a) helping individuals to identify previous and current stressful life situations (major life events and current daily problems) that are antecedents of a negative emotional reaction; (b) minimizing the extent to which such a response impacts negatively on current and future attempts at coping; (c) increasing the effectiveness of problem-solving attempts at coping with current problem situations; and (d) teaching general skills that will enable individuals to deal more effectively with problems in the future to prevent psychological distress.

Depending upon one's idiosyncratic life circumstances, treatment within this context can focus on changing the problematic nature of the antecedent and current stressful life situations, the patient's maladaptive response to these events (through depression and/or substance abuse, or both (5). Problem-solving therapy can be applied in a highly structured, time-limited format similar to our group research programs (11,12), or within a broader, open-ended therapy format. It can be viewed as being the sole treatment program, as part of a larger treatment package, or as a form of maintenance and generalization training. If used in conjunction with other treatment strategies, we recommend that the overall therapy be conducted within a larger, general problem-solving framework (1,4), where the additional techniques are incorporated as a means of facilitating training in a particular problem-solving process. For example, the use of cognitive restructuring would be highly appropriate during problem-definition-and-formulation training to minimize the extent to which various cognitive distortions prevent an individual from accurately defining a problem. Use of relaxation training may also be important during the generation-of-alternatives process to facilitate creativity by decreasing possible interference associated with emotional reactivity, such as anxiety.

B. Problem-Solving Training Components

The following section includes our treatment recommendations for conducting problem-solving therapy for depression. This approach may be specifically applied to a population of depressed individuals who are recovering from an addictive disorder. It is important to note that although this framework appears to be sequentially delineated, actual training should be more flexible and fluid. More specifically, rather than implementing this approach in a static manner, the dynamic interplay among the various components should be highlighted. For example, the use of brainstorming principles can be used throughout training to generate a wide variety of problem-solving goals or a comprehensive list of anticipated consequences instead of during the generation-of-alternatives procedure only.

1. Problem Orientation

This first problem-solving process reflects a general response set involved in understanding and reacting to stressful situations. This orientation can have either a generalized facilitative or inhibiting effect on the remaining four problem-solving tasks. Therefore, actual training in this process is geared toward helping depressed individuals to: (a) correctly identify and recognize problems when they occur; (b) adopt the philosophical perspective that problems in living are normal and inevitable, and that problem solving is a viable means of coping with them; (c) increase their expectations that they are capable of engaging in successful problem-solving activities, that is, their perceived self-efficacy; and (d) inhibit the set to engage in automatic response habits based on previous experiences in similar situations (1,3).

A positive problem orientation would involve acceptance of the beliefs that problems are normal and inevitable, and that one can cope effectively with such problems. To facilitate adopting such an orientation, we recommend the reverse advocacy role-play strategy. According to this technique, the therapist pretends to adopt a particular belief about problems reflective of a negative orientation and asks the patient to provide reasons why that belief is irrational, illogical, incorrect, and/or maladaptive. Such beliefs might include the following statements: "Problems are not common to everyone; if I have a problem, that means that I am crazy!''; "All my problems are caused by me" "There is always a perfect solution to any problem" or "people are not able to change; this is the way that I will always be." At times, when the client has difficulty generating arguments against the therapist's position, the therapist then adopts a more extreme form of the belief, such as "No matter how long it takes, I will continue to try and find the perfect solution to my problem."

If prior clinical assessment indicates that the depressed patient has generalized distortions in information processing, such as negative attributional style, negative appraisals, cognitive distortions, irrational beliefs, then treatment should also be geared to change them. Cognitive restructuring strategies, such as those comprising Beck's (41) cognitive therapy for depression, are recommended in such cases as adjunctive strategies (see Chapter 9).

A second important part of this problem-solving process involves teaching the patient to accurately recognize and label problems when they occur. To facilitate this process, therapists can use various problem checklists (42,43) to help sensitize patients to the array of problems that might occur across a range of areas of life. In addition, patients should also be asked to discuss personal, problematic situations that they have experienced or may experience in their lives, either at work, in friendships, religion, career, finance, relationships, and so on. Problems related to substance abuse are particularly important to identify early on.

Clients are also taught to use feelings or emotions, especially dysphoria, as "cues" or "signals" that a problem exists. We have found it helpful to use visual images of either a traffic stoplight that is flashing red or a waving red flag as signals to "STOP and THINK." Essentially, it is important to teach patients to recognize various situations as problems and to label them as such. Accurately labeling a problem *as* a problem serves to help people to inhibit the tendency to act impulsively or automatically in reaction to the situation.

As part of this training, patients are helped to identify the specific ways they experience emotions in general and depression in particular. This would include physiological arousal and somatic changes, such as feelings of being tired, affective or mood changes, and thoughts such as "I believe that nothing is going to change"). Clients are taught to reframe these reactions from an "overwhelming emotional state of being" to a signal that "something is wrong," just as the red traffic light signals one to "stop and think"). Attention is then redirected to the problem(s) the individual is experiencing with the immediate goal of continuing to engage in the remaining problem-solving tasks.

a. Clinical Example. The following passage is a clinical example of a dialogue between a patient and problem-solving therapist demonstrating the reverse advocacy role-play exercise. Specifically, the client is a 40-year-old salesman, Steve, who abuses alcohol and suffers from depression. He entered treatment several months after he and his wife separated; he has been experiencing feelings of hopelessness and suicidal ideation.

Therapist (TH): Steve, it seems at times that the way you think may have an impact on your feelings. I would like to try a role-play exercise in which I'll take the part of an old friend of yours that you haven't seen in a few months. Just go along with me for now because I'd like to make a certain point. Try your best to make a case against any statements I make that sound irrational or illogical to you, OK?

Patient (P): OK, I'll give it a try.

TH: *(Beginning the role-play)* I know I seem real down lately. I have been a really terrible friend and I wouldn't blame you if you never wanted to talk to me again.

P: What's going on with you? What's wrong?

TH: What's going on? Everything! Absolutely everything! I can't even think of one thing that's going right. My girlfriend has been acting strange lately and I think that she is going to end things with me. Also, my boss reminded me that I have to be evaluated for a raise in the next few weeks. I know for sure that I won't get a raise, and then I'll have to find another job to pay the rent. Forget it. There's no hope for me.

P: Why give up? You have worked hard at your job. You don't know about your girlfriend . . . what's she doing that's so strange?

TH: I don't know. None of my work has paid off. My efforts are pointless. It's all coming down to this . . . disaster.

P: Your efforts are not pointless. A lot of people have rough times at work and you don't know about your girlfriend. Why don't you talk to her? I know how you feel.

TH: But not like this. Don't you know what this means? I definitely won't get the raise. I will have to move out of my apartment. Losing my job and apartment will just make my girlfriend dump me.

P: Look, you don't even know if you're not getting the raise. You don't even have any evidence to say why your girlfriend is leaving you. You don't even sound like you're willing to talk to her. You seem like you're having a rough time right now, but every one has problems like this from time to time. You have to be willing to try to do something about it.

TH: I don't know. This seems worse than anything I have ever seen or heard before.

P: You have to look at this a little differently. First, you need more information about this stuff. You can't come to these conclusions based on what you have told me so far. Anyway, if these things do happen, you'll find a way to get on with your life. Everyone has problems. You are not expected to be perfect.

TH: I feel like I should be perfect and make my boss and my girlfriend happy.

P: It's impossible to be perfect and to never have any problems.

TH: Are you sure about that?

P: Of course I am sure. You have to be realistic. I'm sure that there are some things you can do to help.

b. Clinical Comment. In the preceding example, the therapist presented a problem relevant to the patient's own life experience but focused on a situation that the patient could objectively appraise. The therapist's aim was to strengthen the rational and adaptive attitude that this individual already held concerning failing in interpersonal relationships. The patient should not perceive the clinician as attempting to patronize or mimic his or her beliefs. Rather, the therapist explains that these beliefs at times may engender feelings of distress, which in turn may interfere with later attempts to cope with a stressful problem. The clinician indicates that the purpose of this exercise is to facilitate the patient's adoption of a more positive orientation toward problems in living.

2. Problem Definition and Formulation

The purpose of this first problem-solving task is to understand fully the nature of the problem and to identify a set of realistic goals and objectives. To accomplish this, patients are trained to: (a) seek all available facts and information concerning the problem; (b) describe these facts in clear and unambiguous terms; (c) differentiate relevant from irrelevant information and objective facts from unverified inferences, assumptions, and interpretations; (d) identify the factors and circumstances that make the situation a problem; and (e) set a series of realistic problem-solving goals. In defining and formulating a particular problem, emphasis is placed on accuracy and comprehensiveness.

According to our model, clients are taught to become more systematic and orderly when approaching problems by gathering information, using concrete language, and separating facts from inferences and assumptions. Essentially, individuals learn to ask a wide variety of the five specific "W" questions—*who* ("who is involved in this problem?"; "who is responsible for this problem?"); *what* ("what I am feeling about this problem?"; "what is happening that is making me feel sad?"; "what am I thinking about in reaction to this problem?"; "what will happen if I don't solve this problem?"); *where* ("where is this problem occurring?"); *when* ("when did this problem begin?"; "when am I supposed to solve this problem?"); and *why* ("why did this problem occur?"; "why am I feeling so sad?"). We have found certain occupations to be useful analogies when training patients to use this approach. For example, patients are encouraged to think of themselves in the roles of investigative reporter, detective, or scientist.

In asking these types of questions, the patient is encouraged to use concrete and unambiguous language in order to minimize the likelihood of confusion and distortions of information. Clients are also taught to identify and correct the types of inferences, assumptions, and misconceptions that they might be making while answering these queries (such as selective attention and overgeneralization). Again, various cognitive restructuring strategies can be helpful in this process.

a. Clinical Example. This dialogue will exemplify the importance of separating factual from fictional information when attempting to be an effective problem solver. In the passage provided below, Carolyn, a 30-year-old woman, discusses problems concerning her current feelings of distress. She is happily married with an 11-month-old baby. Her symptoms of depression focused on her feelings of being trapped and conflicted between the demands of motherhood and her eagerness to be a working professional. She had a sense of emptiness and frequently experienced feelings of sadness, guilt, and anger.

Therapist (TH): Let's review the facts you have gathered so far in your attempts to define the main problems you are currently experiencing. Let's look for the information that's most important. Let's also attempt to distinguish between facts and assumptions.

Patient (P): I know I feel really stressed out. I just feel trapped in the house with the baby. Don't get me wrong, I love my baby, but I am starting to envy my husband because he can get out and go to work. He must feel so purposeful. I start to feel angry and depressed in the morning when he is getting ready for work. I do things during the day with my child, and it makes me very happy. I used to work around the clock before I had children and I am not used to this "staying around the house" role.

TH: You mentioned that your husband "must feel so purposeful." Do you feel like what you do is not purposeful?

P: No, I mean I do very important things. Being a mother isn't easy work. The problem is that I feel guilty about wanting to go back to work.

TH: Why not just go back to work and reduce the stress on yourself?

P: Because, I told you, when I am with my baby nothing else matters. I just feel that if I did anything that I enjoy, such as go back to work, that would mean that I am not a good parent.

TH: Is that a fact . . . if you did things that you enjoy that are outside of the demands of being a mother, then that means you are failing as a parent?

P: Well, not really, I mean I would never do anything that I felt would jeopardize the well being of my child. Besides, I guess I do things now that I enjoy. I guess I could even work out of my home when my baby is asleep.

TH: Well, let's not jump ahead and start solving the problem. First, it's important for us to define the problem, and I think that is what we are starting to clear up right now. The problem may not primarily be one of missing your career. Perhaps you have some fears of failing as a parent, and this seems to create a lot of distress for you. Once we have gathered all of the facts and can define this particular problem, then we'll move on to the next task, which is to generate as many ways as we possibly can to solve this particular problem and alleviate some of the distress you are experiencing.

b. Clinical Comment. Although Carolyn originally gathered facts concerning all the areas in her life in which she experienced problems, she had begun to focus on areas that were becoming more salient. It also became clear that Carolyn was making assumptions that were causing her great distress. In fact, when dissecting the problem more carefully, it seemed that her concerns were not based on factual information but on fears and conflicts generated by her newly acquired role. Her problem was eventually defined in terms of reducing the anxiety she experienced regarding her parenting role.

In defining and formulating problems, patients are taught to delineate further specific goals and objectives that they would like to reach. These goals are specified in concrete and unambiguous terms, again, to minimize confusion. Clients are also encouraged to state goals or objectives that are realistic and attainable. It is often the case that a series of subgoals are identified that work as steps to reach the overall problem-solving goal. For example, a client might state that an overall goal is to have a satisfying, long-term relationship with a member of the opposite sex. Important subgoals might include: (a) ameliorating any personal skill deficits, for example, communication problems, that might be contributing to difficulties with relationships; (b) meeting more people in general; (c) dating more frequently; and (d) minimizing the amount of distress associated with disappointments and feelings of rejection when they occur.

In specifying goals, two general types can be identified: *problem-focused goals* and *emotion-focused goals*. Problem-focused goals entail objectives that relate to actual changes in the problem itself. These would be particularly for situations that are possible to change, like getting a new job. On the other hand, emotion-focused goals relate to objectives that are aimed at reducing or minimizing the impact of the distress associated with the experience of a problem. These relate to situations that can be identified as unchangeable, for instance, the death of family member. In most cases, it is likely that both types of goals are important to identify in order to maximize effective problem-solving coping attempts. In the above example, the various subgoals encompass both types of goals.

The last step in problem definition and formulation training involves identifying those obstacles that exist in a given situation that prevent one from reaching specified goals. The factors that make a situation a problem may involve novelty, as when one moves to a new neighborhood, uncertainty, often experienced at the start of a new job, conflicting stimulus demands, which occur in arguments with a spouse over issues of substance abuse, lack of resources, especially limited finances, or some other personal or environmental constraint or deficiency.

In identifying these obstacles, the therapist should be careful to help the patient accurately analyze the problem situation. Often, articulating these obstacles leads to a reevaluation of goals. We have found that several presenting problems of depression that ultimately include goals of increasing one's self-esteem might encompass a variety of subgoals, such as losing weight or improving physical appearance, job skills, and interpersonal relationships. Accurate identification of the obstacles and conflicts involved in a problem helps patients deal better with complex problems and to understand the "real problem."

3. Generation of Alternatives

The overall objective of this component is to make available as many alternative solutions to the problem as possible to increase the likelihood that the most effective ones will eventually be identified. In generating these alternatives, individuals are taught to use three general brainstorming rules: the quantity principle, deferment-of-judgment principle, and variety principle.

According to the quantity principle, the more ideas one produces, the higher the likelihood that effective or good-quality options will be among those generated. Clients are encouraged to produce as many ideas as possible for each of the subgoals (both problem-focused and emotion-focused goals). The second principle, deferment of judgment, suggests that the quantity rule can best be carried out if one withholds judgment about the quality or effectiveness of any idea until an exhaustive list is produced. The only criterion that may be applied is relevance to the problem at hand. Otherwise, evaluation of any option is reserved for the decision-making component.

The last brainstorming rule, the variety principle, encourages individuals to think of a wide range of possible solutions across as many strategies or classes of approaches as possible, instead of focusing only on one or two narrow ideas. In generating solution options, individuals are encouraged to continue to use concrete and umambiguous terms.

a. Clinical Example.   The following is an example of how the generation-of-alternatives task can be implemented in a clinical situation. Albert is a 40-year-old attorney who was a substance abuser with a history of clinical depression. He resigned from his job when he failed to complete an important assignment due to his emotional distress and abuse of alcohol. After completing the clinical assessment, he and his therapist compiled a list of problems that were most pressing for him. One of the items on the list that seemed to be causing Albert the most distress was his unemployment. He was eager to work again but feared that his past failures would impede his ability to find a job. In addition, he seemed unsure whether he wanted to continue his profession as a lawyer.

Therapist (TH): It sounds as though you have been feeling pretty down, and one of the things that has been particularly distressing for you is this problem of wanting to find a job.

Patient (P): Yeah, it is really difficult for me because I know I really messed up with my last job. That stuff goes on record and I can't imagine anyone wanting to hire me. I was really having some problems back then. Nowadays, things are getting better, being in therapy and all, but I don't have a lot of confidence in myself and my abilities anymore.

TH: I see how this is difficult for you. Albert, let's look at the situation a little more closely. You seem to have a lot of distress, with feelings of inadequacy and fear. It might be helpful if we approach this problem and generate the possible alternatives you might use to solve this particular dilemma.

P: I don't think there is any way to solve this. I failed in the past and no one will hire me with my history of quitting due to ah . . . you know . . . mental problems.

TH: I think it might be helpful if at this point we try to keep a positive problem-solving attitude and make a list of all the possibilities. Let's write down as many as we can come up with. Albert, how might you solve this problem of trying to find a job?

P: All I know is the law, criminal law to be exact. I am good at figuring out those who break the law. That is all I am good at.

TH: OK, that's one possibility. Let's write it down.

P: I don't know where you're going with this. That's the only thing I have ever done, and because of my past failure in the career, there is no way I could ever go back. It's no use. This conversation is making me more depressed because it is making me feel more inadequate.

TH: Albert, I wonder if there aren't any other things you are good at or would be willing to learn?

P: I already told you that I don't have any other skills.

TH: I'd like to try an exercise with you that is sometimes quite helpful in situations like this. It's called ''brainstorming.'' It is a technique we use to come up with a lot of possible ways for handling a problem situation so that you can increase your chances of finding a good way of dealing with the problem. First, let's try to come up with as many ideas as possible, and second, let's not worry about how silly an idea might sound. Let's be creative and put off until later judging whether a particular job possibility might be a good one for you.

P: That doesn't make too much sense to me. I could say that I want to be a chef but that's not realistic because I don't know how to cook.

TH: Remember, don't judge your ideas. Let's put that on the list and we'll discuss later how realistic of an option it is for you. What would you need to do to become a chef?

P: I would have to go to culinary school.

TH: Let's put it on the list. You mentioned earlier that you are good at "figuring people out." That sounds like a pretty strong skill to me. What other careers might require you to use that skill?

P: Well, I guess salespeople have to be able to figure out their customers, you know to figure out if they need service or if they would rather be left alone.

TH: That definitely sounds like a relevant option. You're getting the hang of this. What other options might you have?

P: Hmmmm . . . let's see. I guess I could always teach the law. Maybe they would let me in the field if I taught my knowledge to others.

TH: Let's go over what we have so far. Sometimes hearing the others might help us generate additional ideas or combine others that we might not have thought of before. Here's what we have on the list: Criminal Lawyer, Chef, Salesperson, Professor of Law.

P: That's more than I thought we would come up with.

TH: Let's use another brainstorming procedure. It's called the variety principle. What it suggests is that a good list can have several different general strategies for attacking a problem, and that for each general strategy, we should identify several specific tactics or ways of putting the strategy into action. I know this sounds like a lot of information, but let's try it. Which items on the list can be grouped together.

P: Well, two have to do with the law and the others are just different. I would have to go to school to be a chef.

TH: Okay, so one strategy you might have is to find a job related to your knowledge of the law. The tactics you mentioned include teaching or practicing the law. Does this make sense?

P: Yeah, I get it. But, I don't know how I would get a job. I guess I could go to a head hunter, you know one of those people that help you find a job and let them decide.

TH: Sure. Seeking the help of a head hunter would certainly be another strategy to initiate the overall goal of finding a job. Let's add it to the list.

b. Clinical Comment. As illustrated in the preceding example, combining the three principles of brainstorming can lead to both productive and flexible thinking. Albert's initial approach to job finding was pessimistic and quite hopeless. By generating a wide range of possible options not previously identified, he was able to pursue other problem-solving tasks with more optimism and enthusiasm.

4. Design Making

Helping the patient to identify the potential consequences of a particular alternative is an important part of the problem-solving process. This involves generating a list of anticipated outcomes of both short-term and long-term solutions as well as both personal and social consequences.

Personal consequences that can be used as criteria involve the effects of one's emotional well-being, amount of time and effort involved, and effects on one's physical well-being and personal growth. Social outcomes would entail the consequences associated with the well-being of other individuals and their interpersonal relationships with the patient.

In addition, patients are taught to estimate both the likelihood that a given alternative would be effective in reaching their goals and whether they will actually be able to implement the solution optimally, evaluating their unique ability and desire to carry out a solution regardless of its effect on the problem.

Overall, patients learn to evaluate each alternative according to the above major criteria as a means of deciding which alternatives to implement in real life. The overall cost-benefit ratio for each coping option can be calculated according to a simple rating scale (for example,

-3 = *very unsatisfactory* to $+3$ = *very satisfactory*). An idea that appears to have a large number of positive consequences and a minimal amount of cost might be rated as $+2$ or $+3$. Conversely, an alternative that is expected to yield few positive outcomes and a large number of negative consequences would be rated as -2 or -3.

Using these ratings, individuals may then develop an overall solution plan by first comparing the ratings of the various alternative solutions. If only a small number of ideas appear to be rated as potentially satisfactory, then the problem solver must ask several evaluative questions: "Do I have enough information?"; "Did I define the problem correctly?"; "Are my goals too high?"; "Did I generate enough options?" At this point, the patient may need to go back and engage again in the previous problem-solving tasks.

If several effective or satisfactory alternatives are identified, then the patient is encouraged to include a combination of potentially effective coping options for each subgoal to "attack" the problem from a variety of perspectives. Further, a contingency plan complete with alternative coping options is often useful in the event the first group of options fails.

    a.   Clinical Example.   Harriet is a 55-year-old woman who was recently diagnosed with breast cancer. Since the diagnosis, Harriet had experienced clinical symptoms of depression that were unrelated to the medical procedures. In working with Harriet, we discovered that her fears of being ill or dying were accompanied by additional concerns. Harriet is a widow, living alone, with her adult children nearby. Wanting to remain independent and strong, however, she minimized her need for visitors and support from her friends and family. Respecting her needs, her loved ones made a sincere effort to give Harriet her space during her recovery. During therapy, this problem was defined as "wanting to have loved ones in her company more often."

During several brainstorming sessions, the following alternative solutions were generated by the patient:

1.   Request that others visit by writing them a letter.
2.   Buy a pet.
3.   Have a party.
4.   Visit others when feeling well.

5. Invite her family to a session so we can problem solve as a team.
6. Go to the local community center and see if volunteers can come to my home.
7. Talk to my friends and family and ask them to visit more often.
8. Meet new people and forget my family.

The sessions focusing on decision making involved evaluating these suggested alternatives. During these sessions, Harriet has already begun to rate each alternative for the likelihood of meeting her desired goals.

Therapist (TH): Let's review and rate the solutions you have come up with in terms of the likelihood of meeting your goals. You can immediately disregard those that are very unlikely for you Harriet.

Patient (P): Well, I would rather not forget my family. I would much rather try those that get them back in my life and let them know how much I need them.

TH: Okay. Let's start with the first option, which involves writing your family and friends a letter, telling them your feelings, and requesting that they visit more often. How likely would this alternative be in helping meet your primary goal?

P: Well, it would give them the message, but they might be hurt that I wasn't comfortable telling them to their face. Give that a "1."

TH: Do you think this alternative would overcome some of the obstacles we mentioned earlier, such as feelings of wanting to remain independent?

P: No, not unless I stated in the letter that I need them but not too much. I miss their company, and I need them sometimes to get around the house, but I still want my space and for them to go on with their lives. I'll give that a "1" too.

TH: What about the obstacle of feeling lonely?

P: Well, if they visited more often as a result of my letter then that would be wonderful. When you put it that way I have to give it a "2."

TH: Good work, Harriet. Do you see how just in examining goals and obstacles, you can see that the same alternative can have several different ratings?

P: Yes.

TH: What about the next alternative of buying a pet.

P: Well, I have to laugh. Although a pet would make me feel less lonely, I still need to get my family and friends back in my life. I can only give that alternative a "1."

TH: You are really getting the hang of this, Harriet. Let's keep going.

   b. Clinical Comment. During this session, Harriet appears to have been able to engage in a systematic evaluation of each alternative, targeting one criterion at a time. At this point, it is important to reinforce the development of this skill, while continuing to acknowledge the presence of habituated, emotionalizing past ways of coping as predictable and acceptable.

5. *Solution Implementation and Verification*

The first part of the last problem-solving task involves the performance of the chosen solution options. The second aspect entails the careful monitoring and evaluation of the actual solution outcomes. After the solution plan is carried out, individuals are encouraged to monitor the real-life consequences that occur as a function of the implemented solution. Clients are taught to develop self-monitoring methods that are relevant to a given problem that would include: (a) ratings of the solution outcome itself (Did the plan achieve the specified goals? What were the positive consequences? What were the negative consequences?); (b) evaluative ratings of one's emotional reactions to these outcomes (How do I feel about these outcomes? Do they make me happy? Am I less anxious?); and the degree to which outcomes match the consequences previously anticipated during the decision-making process (Did what I predict was going to happen actually happen?) If the match is satisfactory, then the problem solver is encouraged to administer some form of self-reinforcement, such as self-statements of congratulation or a tangible gift or reward. On the other hand, if the match is unsatisfactory, then he or she is encouraged to either implement the previously identified contingency plan or to recycle through the entire problem-solving process. Particular care should be exercised to differentiate between difficulties with the *performance* or implementation of a coping option and the problem-solving *process* itself.

a. Clinical Example. Don was a recent patient who responded well to the earlier parts of problem-solving training. However, when it was time to actually implement his solution plan, he remained hesitant, fearing that he would be unable to cope effectively. At this time, it was appropriate to reintroduce concepts that were initially discussed during problem orientation, the first part of the training. Secondly, Don was encouraged to use a comparison worksheet, a procedure useful to this stage of the problem-solving process. This worksheet asked Don to list a variety of possible outcomes that might occur if the problem remained unsolved. In addition, he was asked to make a list of potential consequences if the best alternative was actually carried out. The following demonstrates the completion of this exercise.

Therapist (TH): OK, Don. Last session I requested that you complete the worksheet I gave you. Did you have a chance to do it this week?

Patient (P): I tried listing some of the consequences that might happen if I don't solve the problem of communicating with my girlfriend, right?

TH: Absolutely. It's important to think and list both the positive and negative consequences that will occur if the problem is or is not solved. Tell me what you came up with.

P: Well, I guess if I don't talk to her about our problems, I am still going to feel miserable about myself and my performance at work will still suffer.

TH: So, one of the possible consequences involves a negative evaluation. Is that right?

P: Yeah . . . I really will feel terrible if I don't do something about this soon.

TH: Have you identified any other consequences?

P: Well, I have thought a whole lot about how much better things would be if I were able to work things out with my girlfriend. I would feel better about myself and certainly do a better job at work. In fact, if I do well at work, I will have enough money to buy my girlfriend something special for her birthday.

TH: It sounds as if you have been thinking about this a lot, and that there are lots of positive things in store if you are able to solve this problem.

P: Yeah . . . I am ready to do it. I can't be afraid of confronting our problems anymore. Like you always remind me, problems are normal, everyone has problems. It's time I did something about this so I can start feeling better about myself.

b. Clinical Comment.   In the preceding illustration, Don, in comparing the possible consequences of solving the problem with *not* solving the problem, became more optimistic and motivated to implement his solution plan. This exercise can facilitate movement toward overcoming motivational difficulties or fears of failure. It may be important for the therapist to initially address subgoals that have a higher probability of being reached to provide for a reinforcing experience early in treatment. This shaping procedure is especially relevant for depressed individuals with strong beliefs of poor self-efficacy.

It is possible that behavioral skills deficits may prevent the individual from implementing a solution in its optimal form. It is important to evaluate alternatives during the decision-making process to estimate the likelihood that the patient will be able to carry out a particular solution optimally.

VI.   IMPORTANT GENERAL
CLINICAL CONSIDERATIONS

In addition to the specific training guidelines just provided, we offer a set of general clinical considerations or hints concerning the optimal implementation of problem-solving therapy.

1. In addition to providing didactic explanations of each of the various components of the overall problem-solving approach, therapists should also *model* or demonstrate the manner in which they can be used.
2. As many real-life and patient-relevant problems as possible should be used as examples to illustrate the various components.
3. Therapists should be careful not to present this approach as a cold, rational, or sterile process of thinking. Many clients initially react to this approach as either too simplistic (''I don't have any difficulties solving financial or job problems. I thought we

were going to focus on my deep-seated problems") or "cold" ("How can I try to be so rational when I feel unhappy?"). In addition, symptoms of lethargy, anhedonia, and decreased motivation require the use of initial strategies designed to mobilize a patient toward at least minimally active participation. For example, clients need a thorough understanding of the complexities of this model and its underlying assumptions to provide a framework from which they can understand how difficulties in coping with stressful situations can lead to depression and repeated abuse of alcohol and drugs (1). Moreover, providing a detailed analysis of a given client's problems and associated depression helps to minimize these initial negative reactions. Further, conceptualizing such reactions within the problem-orientation process and illustrating how such reactions may inhibit effective coping attempts also helps to minimize impulsive rejections of this model. Last, it maybe helpful to indicate to the patient that the problem-solving process is largely the way therapists themselves think about finding answers to problems (44). Clients, ultimately, are trained to become their own "therapists."

4. If at any time later in treatment, patients seem to harbor feelings of incompetency with regard to their ability to solve problems effectively or to view problems as catastrophic, *problem orientation exercises should be reintroduced.* It is hoped that by reviewing this step, a positive and optimistic attitude toward problem solving will be recaptured.

5. Patients should be encouraged to complete various homework assignments between sessions that address a particular problem-solving task (for instance, generating solutions to a problem experienced that week, implementing a solution plan that had been developed during a session) as a means of increasing generalization and maintenance.

6. Behavioral rehearsal of the various problem-solving tasks should be emphasized throughout training. Although individuals may be able to learn these problem-solving coping strategies, it is important that frequent opportunities for practicing these skills are provided. Therapists should include opportunities for the

actual implementation of various solutions during treatment so that clients may experience engaging in the entire problem-solving process and in particular, in successful problem resolution.

7. Therapists should emphasize the difference between *problem-focused coping* and *emotion-focused coping*. Problem-focused coping involves attempts to change the nature of the situation itself. Emotion-focused coping attempts are geared toward changing one's emotional reactions to a problem. In real-life situations, it is often impossible to have complete control over all situations. For example, the loss of a loved one engenders significant grief and depressive reactions that are normal. To suggest that the problem can be solved by replacing the loved one misses the appropriate therapeutic mark by far.

VII. SUMMARY REMARKS

We began this chapter by defining the constructs of social problem solving, problematic situations, solutions, and effective solutions. Our model of problem-solving therapy for depression is based heavily on the approach originally delineated by D'Zurilla and Goldfried and later revised by D'Zurilla and Nezu. We offered several methods by which clinicians can both assess problem-solving deficits as well as improvements in such deficits that can occur as a function of training. These include the Problem Solving Inventory, the revised version of the Social Problem-Solving Inventory, and the Means-End Problem-Solving procedure.

An abbreviated manual outlining treatment recommendations for conducting problem-solving therapy was then presented. Training exercises were included for each of the five problem-solving processes (problem orientation, problem definition and formulation, generation of alternatives, decision making, solution implementation and verification). Last, a variety of additional clinical recommendations were offered to facilitate optimal implementation of this approach.

We conclude this chapter with a quote from an address by John F. Kennedy to American University on June 10, 1963 to underscore a positive problem orientation: ''No problem of human destiny is beyond human beings.''

REFERENCES

1. A. M. Nezu, C. M. Nezu, and M. G. Perri, *Problem-Solving Therapy for Depression: Theory, Research, and Clinical Guidelines,* Wiley, New York, 1989.
2. T. J. D'Zurilla, and M. R. Goldfried, *J. Abnormal Psychology 78:*107–126 (1971).
3. T. J. D'Zurilla, and A. M. Nezu, *Advances in Cognitive-Behavioral Research and Therapy* (P. C. Kendall, ed.), Academic Press, New York, 1982, pp. 201–274.
4. T. J. D'Zurilla, *Problem-Solving Therapy: A Social Competence Approach to Clinical Intervention,* Springer, New York, 1986.
5. A. M. Nezu, *Clinical Psychology Review 7:*121–144 (1987).
6. A. M. Nezu, and T. J. D'Zurilla, *Anxiety and Depression: Distinctive and Overlapping Features* (P. C. Kendall, and D. Watson, eds.), Academic Press, New York, 1989, pp. 285–315.
7. T. J. D'Zurilla, and A. Maydeau-Olivares, Manuscript submitted for publication.
8. P. P. Heppner, *The Problem Solving Inventory,* Consulting Psychologists Press, Palo Alto, CA 1988.
9. T. J. D'Zurilla, and A. Maydeau-Olivares, Manuscript submitted for publication.
10. T. J. D'Zurilla, and A. M. Nezu, *Psychological Assessment: J. Consult. Clin. Psychol. 2:*156–163 (1990).
11. A. M. Nezu, *J. Consult. Clin. Psychol. 54:*196–202 (1986)
12. A. M. Nezu, and M. G. Perri, *J. Consult. Clin. Psychol. 57:*408–413 (1989).
13. P. A. Arean, M. G. Perri, A. M. Nezu, R. L. Schein, F. Christopher, and T. X. Joseph, *J. Consult. Clin. Psychol. 61:*1003–1010 (1993).
14. J. J. Platt, and G. Spivack, *Manual for the Means-End Problem-Solving Procedure (MEPS): A Measure of Interpersonal Cognitive Problem-Solving Skills,* Hahnemann University, Philadelphia, 1975.
15. P. C. Kendall, and G. L. Fischler, *Child Dev. 55:*879–892 (1984).
16. I. H. Gotlib, and R. F. Asarnow, *J. Consult. Clin. Psychol. 47:*86–95 (1979).
17. A. M. and Nezu, G. F. Ronan, *The Southern Psychologist 3:*29–34 (1987).

18. A. M. Nezu, *J. Counseling Psychology 32:*135–138 (1985).

19. A. T. Beck, C. H. Ward, M. Mendelsohn, J. Mock, and J. Erbaugh, *Arch. Gen. Psychiatry 5:*462–476 (1961).

20. P. P. Heppner, and W. P. Anderson, *Cognitive Therapy and Research 9:*415–427 (1985).

21. A. M. Nezu, *J. Clin. Psychol. 42:*42–49 (1986).

22. American Psychiatric Association, *Diagnostic and Statistical Manual of Mental Disorders* (3rd ed.), Washington, DC, 1980.

23. E. M. Marx, J. M. G. Williams, and G. C. Claridge, *J. Abnormal Psychology* 101:78–86, (1992).

24. L. A. Doerfler, and C. S. Richards, *Cognitive Therapy and Research 5:*237–249 (1981).

25. E. E. Beckham, and R. L. Adams, *Behav. Res. Ther. 22:*71–75 (1984).

26. A. M. Nezu, and G. F. Ronan, *J. Consult. Clin. Psychol. 53:*693–697 (1985).

27. A. M. Nezu, *J. Clin. Psychol. 42:*847–852 (1986).

28. A. M. Nezu, C. M. Nezu, L. Saraydarian, K. Kalmar, and G. F. Ronan, *Cognitive Therapy and Research 10:*489–498 (1986).

29. P. P. Heppner, M. Kampa, and L. Brunning, *Cognitive Therapy and Research 11:*155–168 (1984).

30. A. M. Nezu, and G. F. Ronan, *J. Counseling Psychology 35:*134–138 (1988).

31. C. M. Nezu, A. M. Nezu, and P. A. Arean, *Research in Developmental Disabilities 12:*371–386 (1992).

32. R. A. Hussian, and P. S. Lawrence, *Cognitive Therapy and Research 5:*57–69 (1981).

33. K. J. Sher, *Psychological Theories of Drinking and Alcoholism* (H. T. Blane, and K. E. Leonard, eds.), Guilford Press, New York, 1987, pp. 227–271.

34. J. J. Platt, D. O. Taube, D. S. Metzger, and M. J. Duome, *J. Cognitive Psychotherapy 2:*5–34 (1988).

35. J. G. Williams, and K. J. Kleinfelter, *Psychological Reports 65:*1235–1244 (1989).

36. K. B. Carey, and M. P. Carey, *J. Psychopathology and Behavioral Assessment 12:*247–154 (1990).

37. S. J. Nixon, R. Tivis, and O. A. Parsons, *Alcoholism: Clinical and Experimental Research 16:*684–687 (1992).

38. J. Intagliatia, *J. Consult. Clin. Psychol. 46:*489–498 (1978).

39. H. Getter, M. D. Litt, R. M. Kadden, and N. L. Cooney, *Int. J. Group Psychother. 42:*419–430 (1992).

40. M. J. Elias, M. A. Gara, T. F. Schuyler, L. R. Branden-Muller, and M. A. Sayette. *Amer. J. Orthopsychiatry 61:*409–417 (1991).
41. A. T. Beck, A. J. Rush, B. F. Shaw, and G. Emery, *Cognitive Therapy of Depression: A Treatment Manual,* Guilford Press, New York 1979.
42. R. L. Mooney, and L. V. Gordon, *Manual: The Mooney Problem Checklist,* Psychological Corporation, New York 1950.
43. J. A. Schinka, *Personal Problems Checklist,* Psychological Corporation, Odessa, FL 1986.
44. (A. M. Nezu, and C. M. Nezu, eds.), *Clinical decision making in behavior therapy: A problem-solving approach,* Research Press, Champaign, IL, 1992.

Index

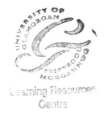

About the Editor

Jerry S. Kantor is Medical Director of the Addiction Recovery Centre, Fort Myers, Florida. A Diplomate of the American Board of Psychiatry, Dr. Kantor is the author or coauthor of numerous professional publications and a reviewer for the *American Journal of Psychiatry*. He serves on the editorial board of the *American Journal of Drug and Alcohol Abuse* (Marcel Dekker, Inc.) and is a member of the American Psychiatric Association and the American Academy of Psychiatrists in Alcoholism and Addictions. Dr. Kantor attended the University of Houston, Texas, and the University of San Francisco, California, as an undergraduate, and received the M.D. degree (1974) from the University of Texas Medical Branch at Galveston. He did his residency training in psychiatry at New York Hospital-Cornell Medical Center, Westchester Division.